Built From Fat

Why Your Body Runs on Structure, Not Calories

First Edition: March 2026
ISBN: 978-1-966035-04-6
Published by Elite Nutrition Research
EliteNutritionResearch.com

ELITE

NUTRITION RESEARCH

Elite Nutrition Research is a science-driven health and education company dedicated to understanding and optimizing human physiology at its most fundamental level. Our work is built on an architecture-first approach—examining how nutrients interact with cellular systems, membranes, energy production, and signaling pathways to shape overall health and performance. Rather than following trends, we focus on first principles, combining biochemical insight, formulation precision, and practical application to create both advanced nutritional products and in-depth educational systems.

Through our books, courses, and formulations, Elite Nutrition Research aims to give individuals direct access to the mechanisms that govern their biology—empowering them to think clearly, act intentionally, and build lasting health from the inside out.

To explore our full system of products, courses, and research, visit:
www.elitenutritionresearch.com

Table of Contents

INTRODUCTION

THE GREAT BIOLOGICAL MISUNDERSTANDING

Modern nutrition did not lose its way through a lack of data. It lost its structure. Once the body was reduced to an energy-processing system, food was stripped of its physical meaning and recast as interchangeable fuel. Fat, carbohydrate, and protein were assigned values based on combustion rather than function, and from that point forward, the material differences between them were treated as secondary. The body became an accounting problem. Inputs were measured, outputs were estimated, and the internal machinery was assumed to behave predictably as long as the numbers balanced. That assumption removed the one variable that actually determines behavior: what the body is built from.

The human organism is not defined by how much energy it processes. It is defined by how it is constructed. Every cell maintains a boundary that separates internal chemistry from the external environment while allowing controlled exchange. That boundary is not theoretical. It is a lipid structure with measurable physical properties. Its composition determines how easily ions pass, how tightly gradients are held, how receptors behave, and how signals move across space and time. When the composition of that boundary changes, those properties change with it. Electrical stability shifts. Signal timing drifts. Transport becomes either restricted or excessive. None of this is captured by calorie models because energy does not define structure. Structure determines how energy is used, where it is directed, and whether it produces stable output or systemic noise.

When lipids were reclassified as fuel, their role as structural material was ignored. Dietary fat became something to burn or store, not something to build with. This created a mismatch between input and requirement. The body continued to rely on lipids to construct membranes, organize signaling domains, and stabilize electrical systems, but the incoming material became increasingly inconsistent in quality and composition. Over time, this forces continuous remodeling under suboptimal conditions. Membranes lose coherence. Receptors fail to maintain consistent orientation. Signaling pathways activate without clean termination. The system compensates, but compensation has limits, and once those limits are reached, instability begins to spread across systems that appear unrelated but share the same underlying structure.

Inflammation, in this context, is not an isolated response. It is the consequence of structural disturbance within membranes that alters how signals are generated and resolved. Hormonal instability follows the same pattern. Receptors embedded in unstable lipid environments do not respond predictably, even when hormone levels are unchanged. Metabolic dysfunction emerges when mitochondrial membranes lose the ability to maintain tight gradients, forcing energy production to become inefficient and inconsistent. These outcomes are often treated as separate conditions, each with its own explanation, but they are better understood as different expressions of the same architectural problem.

Energy-based thinking cannot resolve this because it operates at the wrong level of the system. A calorie can describe potential input, but it does not determine whether a membrane will hold its structure under stress, whether a receptor will cluster correctly, or whether a signal will propagate with precision. It cannot explain why two individuals consuming the same amount of energy can produce entirely different physiological outcomes. Those differences arise from how the system is built, not how much fuel it receives.

Reframing the body as a lipid-structured system changes how inputs are evaluated. Dietary fat is no longer a passive energy source. It is a material that integrates into membranes over time, altering their physical properties and, by extension, the behavior of every system that depends on them. Some lipids reinforce stability, resist oxidative damage, and support consistent signaling. Others introduce fragility, increase susceptibility to breakdown, and amplify noise within the system. These effects are not immediate in the way energy is. They accumulate through repeated incorporation and remodeling, gradually shifting the operating characteristics of the organism.

This shift in perspective removes the need to treat symptoms as isolated failures. When structure is corrected, function follows without direct intervention at every downstream point. Membranes regain consistency. Signaling becomes coherent. Energy production stabilizes because the conditions required for it are restored. The body does not need to be forced into balance. It returns to balance when the materials used to build it support stable operation.

The central error, then, is not simply that fat was misunderstood. It is that the body was mischaracterized as an energy system rather than a structural system. Once that error is corrected, the rest of the model begins to align. Food is no longer evaluated by how much energy it provides, but by what it becomes. Physiology is no longer explained through isolated pathways, but through the behavior of interconnected structures. The outcomes that once appeared complex begin to resolve into predictable patterns because they are governed by physical constraints rather than abstract models.

The Collapse of Structure into Calories

The reduction of food to calories replaced physical reality with abstraction. Once energy became the dominant lens, the material differences between fats, carbohydrates, and proteins were treated as secondary details rather than primary determinants of biological behavior. Combustion values became the organizing principle. Four calories per gram for carbohydrate, nine for fat, and the system was considered explained. This framing removed the question of what these substances become once they enter the body and replaced it with how much energy they could theoretically release. The body was modeled as a furnace instead of a constructed system, and in that transition, the role of structure disappeared from the equation.

This shift did not occur because it accurately described physiology, but because it simplified measurement. Energy can be quantified cleanly. Structure cannot. Membrane composition, receptor organization, lipid domain behavior, and electrical stability do not reduce to a single number. They require a layered model that accounts for physical arrangement, material properties, and dynamic interaction over time. By abandoning that complexity, nutrition gained simplicity at the cost of accuracy. Foods that produce identical caloric values were treated as equivalent inputs, even though they deliver entirely different structural materials that integrate into the body in distinct ways.

When structure is removed from the model, cause and effect become obscured. A system built from unstable lipid inputs will behave differently from one built from stable materials, even if total caloric intake is identical. Membranes assembled from highly unsaturated fatty acids exhibit increased susceptibility to oxidative damage, altered permeability, and inconsistent receptor behavior. These changes propagate outward. Ion gradients become less stable. Signal transduction becomes noisy. Mitochondrial efficiency declines as membrane integrity weakens. None of these effects can be predicted by caloric value because they are not functions of energy quantity. They are functions of material composition.

The calorie model also fails to account for time. Structural integration is not immediate. Dietary lipids are absorbed, transported, and gradually incorporated into cellular membranes through continuous remodeling cycles. Each cycle replaces a portion of existing structure with new material. Over weeks and months, this process shifts the physical properties of tissues. A system repeatedly supplied with unstable inputs will accumulate instability. A system supplied with stable inputs will move toward coherence. Energy accounting captures none of this because it treats each intake event as isolated rather than cumulative.

Once energy became the dominant framework, interventions followed the same logic. Reducing fat intake was interpreted as reducing energy density, without considering that this also reduces the availability of structural materials required to maintain membrane integrity. Replacing those fats with carbohydrates preserved caloric intake while altering the composition of the system being built. The body continued to assemble itself, but with different inputs, leading to predictable changes in behavior that were then labeled as new conditions rather than recognized as consequences of altered structure.

The collapse into calories also created a disconnect between measurement and outcome. Individuals consuming similar caloric amounts can produce entirely different physiological states because their internal structures differ. One system may maintain stable membranes, coherent signaling, and efficient energy production, while another operates with degraded boundaries, erratic signaling, and constant compensatory stress. The calorie model cannot explain this divergence because it does not measure the variables that drive it.

Reintroducing structure into the model resolves this gap. Food is not an abstract source of energy. It is a set of materials that enter the body, integrate into its architecture, and alter its behavior over time. Lipids in particular do not pass through the system unchanged. They become the system. They define the properties of membranes, the behavior of receptors, and the stability of energy production. When this is accounted for, outcomes that appeared inconsistent begin to follow predictable patterns. Systems built from stable materials behave in stable ways. Systems built from unstable materials require constant compensation and eventually lose coherence.

The mistake was not in measuring energy, but in allowing that measurement to replace the underlying reality it was meant to describe. Calories can quantify potential, but they cannot define function. Function emerges from structure, and once structure is removed from the model, the system becomes impossible to predict with any precision.Lipids reclassified as fuel instead of material

Why Energy Models Fail to Predict Biological Behavior

Energy models treat the body as a system defined by input and output, where biological outcomes are expected to follow from the balance between what enters and what is expended. This assumes that the internal machinery behaves consistently regardless of what it is built from. In practice, the machinery itself is variable. Cells do not process energy in a uniform environment. They operate within membranes whose composition determines permeability, electrical resistance, receptor behavior, and transport dynamics. When those properties shift, the same amount of energy entering the system produces different results because it is being processed under different physical conditions.

A calorie does not specify how energy is handled once it reaches the cell. It does not determine whether glucose transporters are properly positioned within the membrane, whether insulin receptors can cluster and signal efficiently, or whether mitochondrial membranes can maintain the gradients required for controlled energy production. These are structural variables. When membrane composition becomes unstable, transport becomes inconsistent. Substrates either fail to enter efficiently or enter without proper regulation. This creates oscillation in availability, forcing the system to compensate through hormonal adjustments that appear as dysregulation rather than a predictable response to altered structure.

Mitochondrial function exposes the limits of energy-based thinking more clearly. ATP production depends on the ability of the inner mitochondrial membrane to maintain a proton gradient. That gradient is a physical separation held by the integrity of the membrane itself. If the membrane becomes permeable due to lipid instability or oxidative damage, protons leak across it. The system responds by increasing electron flow in an attempt to maintain output, which raises reactive oxygen production and further degrades the structure. Energy is still entering the system, but it is no longer being converted efficiently because the conditions required for controlled conversion are no longer present. A calorie-based model cannot account for this because it does not include gradient stability as a variable.

Signal timing is another dimension that energy models do not capture. Hormonal signaling depends on receptors embedded within lipid environments that determine how signals are initiated, amplified, and terminated. When membranes lose organization, receptor behavior becomes inconsistent. Signals may initiate without proper amplification or persist longer than intended due to delayed termination. This produces overlapping signaling states, where multiple pathways remain active simultaneously, creating noise within the system. The energy entering the system has not changed, but the interpretation of that energy at the cellular level has become distorted.

The model also fails to account for how energy demand is generated. Demand is not fixed. It is influenced by the stability of the system itself. When membranes are compromised, ion gradients leak, requiring constant correction. The cell expends energy not for productive work, but to maintain basic separation. This increases baseline energy consumption without improving output. Two systems receiving identical caloric input can diverge because one is spending energy maintaining unstable structure while the other is directing energy toward functional processes. The difference is not in the quantity of energy, but in how much of it is lost to maintaining compromised architecture.

Time further separates energy models from biological reality. Structural changes accumulate gradually as membranes are remodeled with incoming materials. This alters system behavior long before changes in energy intake occur. A system can move toward instability while caloric intake remains constant because the materials being integrated are shifting the properties of the structure itself. By the time measurable outcomes appear, the underlying architecture has already changed.

Energy models interpret these outcomes as imbalances in input or output, when they are the result of altered structural conditions that were never measured.

Energy accounting provides a narrow view that can describe how much enters and how much leaves, but it does not explain how the system behaves in between. Biological behavior emerges from the interaction between structure and input, not from input alone. Without accounting for membrane composition, signaling organization, and gradient stability, predictions based on energy remain incomplete. The same input can produce different outcomes because the system processing that input is not constant. Once structure is included, variability becomes predictable. Without it, outcomes appear inconsistent and are attributed to factors that do not address the underlying cause.

The Return to Structure as the Primary Model

Reintroducing structure restores the missing variable that connects input to outcome. The body is not an abstract processor of energy but a material system assembled from specific components that determine how every process behaves. Once this is recognized, the question shifts from how much energy enters the system to what physical conditions exist inside it. Membranes define those conditions. Their composition sets permeability, electrical resistance, receptor organization, and the stability of gradients that drive transport and energy production. When these properties are consistent, inputs are handled predictably. When they are not, the same inputs produce variable and often unstable outcomes.

Structure establishes the rules under which all biochemical reactions occur. Enzymes do not operate in isolation. Their activity depends on orientation, proximity to substrates, and the surrounding environment, all of which are influenced by membrane state. Receptors require organized lipid domains to bind ligands and transmit signals with precision. When those domains lose coherence, signaling becomes fragmented. Inputs still arrive, but they are interpreted differently because the physical context has changed. This is why restoring structure precedes any attempt to correct downstream processes. Without stable architecture, interventions act on shifting ground and produce inconsistent results.

The return to structure also redefines how time is understood in physiology. Structural change is cumulative. Lipids introduced through diet are incorporated into membranes through continuous remodeling, gradually altering their properties. This process does not produce immediate shifts in the way energy intake does, but it changes the operating characteristics of the system over longer intervals. As membranes are rebuilt with more stable materials, permeability tightens, receptor behavior stabilizes, and gradients become easier to maintain. The system begins to require less compensatory effort to sustain basic function, and energy can be directed toward productive work rather than constant correction.

This framework resolves the apparent disconnect between similar inputs and different outcomes. Two individuals consuming comparable amounts of energy can produce different physiological states because their internal structures are not equivalent. One system may be built from materials that support stable membranes and coherent signaling, while another is assembled from components that degrade under stress and require continuous repair. The difference is not explained by energy balance. It is explained by the condition of the structure processing that energy. Once structure is measured and addressed, variability becomes predictable rather than arbitrary.

Returning to structure changes how intervention is approached. Instead of attempting to force outcomes through isolated adjustments, the focus shifts to rebuilding the conditions that allow the system to regulate itself. Stable lipid inputs replace unstable ones. Oxidative pressure is reduced so membranes can maintain integrity. Signaling pathways regain clarity because the environments that support them are restored. This does not act as a direct correction of every symptom. It alters the underlying conditions that produce those symptoms, allowing multiple systems to realign simultaneously because they share the same structural foundation.

In this model, nutrients are evaluated by what they become within the system rather than by their immediate effects. Lipids are not consumed for energy alone. They are incorporated into membranes where they influence behavior continuously. Some reinforce stability and resist degradation, supporting consistent signaling and energy production. Others introduce fragility, increasing susceptibility to breakdown and amplifying noise within the system. These differences accumulate over time through repeated incorporation, gradually shifting the operating state of the organism.

The return to structure does not discard energy. It places it in context. Energy remains necessary, but it is no longer treated as the primary determinant of function. It is a resource that must be processed within a defined architecture. When that architecture is stable, energy is used efficiently and predictably. When it is unstable, energy is diverted toward maintaining basic conditions rather than producing useful work. By restoring structure as the primary model, the body becomes understandable again because its behavior follows from physical constraints that can be observed, influenced, and rebuilt.

PART I

THE LIPID FOUNDATION OF HUMAN STRUCTURE

Chapter 1

The Body as a Lipid System

The human body is organized around boundaries. Every function, from cellular metabolism to whole-system coordination, depends on the ability to maintain separation between internal and external environments while allowing controlled exchange. This separation is not conceptual. It is built from lipids. Each cell is enclosed by a membrane composed primarily of phospholipids, cholesterol, and embedded proteins, forming a dynamic structure that defines what enters, what exits, and how signals are transmitted. Without this boundary, gradients collapse, signaling fails, and the distinction between inside and outside disappears. The body does not begin with energy. It begins with containment.

Membranes do more than enclose. Their composition determines how the system behaves under load. The arrangement of lipid tails affects fluidity, which in turn controls how proteins embedded in the membrane can move, interact, and function. Cholesterol modulates this environment by stabilizing the membrane, preventing excessive rigidity at low temperatures and excessive permeability at high temperatures. These properties are not static. They shift continuously based on the materials available to the system. When lipid composition changes, the behavior of the membrane changes with it. Permeability alters. Electrical resistance shifts. The ability to hold ion gradients either strengthens or weakens. These changes propagate outward, affecting every process that depends on stable separation.

Electrical stability emerges directly from membrane integrity. Cells maintain differences in ion concentration across their membranes, creating gradients that store potential energy. This stored potential drives nerve impulses, muscle contraction, and transport processes throughout the body. If the membrane becomes too permeable, ions leak across it, forcing the cell to expend energy to restore balance. This constant correction increases baseline demand while reducing efficiency. The system begins to operate under strain, not because energy is lacking, but because structure no longer holds the conditions required for efficient use.

Signal transmission depends on organized lipid environments. Receptors are not randomly distributed across the membrane. They cluster within specific regions where lipid composition supports their function. These microdomains allow signals to be initiated, amplified, and terminated with precision. When membrane composition becomes unstable, these domains lose coherence. Receptors drift, clustering becomes inconsistent, and signaling pathways activate without proper coordination. The result is not simply reduced signaling, but distorted signaling, where messages are initiated, prolonged, or terminated incorrectly. The system receives input, but the interpretation of that input becomes unreliable.

The body extends this lipid architecture across multiple scales. Organelles within the cell are also defined by membranes, each with distinct compositions tailored to their function. The mitochondrion relies on a tightly controlled inner membrane to maintain the gradients required for energy production. The endoplasmic reticulum uses its membrane structure to synthesize and process lipids and proteins. Vesicles transport materials by merging and separating membranes in controlled sequences. At the tissue level, cells coordinate through membrane interactions, forming barriers, junctions, and communication networks that maintain system-wide organization. This continuity reveals a single principle repeated across scales: function follows from how boundaries are constructed and maintained.

Dietary lipids feed directly into this architecture. They are absorbed, transported, and incorporated into membranes through ongoing remodeling processes. This integration is not selective in a way that filters out all variability. The materials available influence what is built. If the incoming lipids are stable and resistant to degradation, membranes move toward greater coherence. If they are prone to oxidation or structural instability, those characteristics become part of the system. Over time, this alters how cells behave, how signals are processed, and how energy is managed. The body is not insulated from its inputs. It is continuously rebuilt from them.

Viewing the body as a lipid system resolves inconsistencies that arise under energy-based models. It explains why identical caloric intake can produce different outcomes, why signaling becomes unreliable under certain dietary conditions, and why restoring stability often requires changes in material input rather than adjustments in energy balance. The system is not reacting unpredictably. It is expressing the properties of the structure it is built from. When that structure is stable, behavior becomes consistent. When it is not, variability emerges as a direct consequence of degraded boundaries.

This framework establishes the foundation for understanding physiology as a function of material composition. Lipids are not a secondary component of the system. They are the medium through which the system exists and operates. Every subsequent process, from signaling to energy production, is constrained by the properties of this medium. To understand how the body functions, it must first be understood as a system built from lipids, where boundaries define behavior and structure determines outcome.

The Body as a Boundary-Defined System

The body operates by maintaining separation. Every function depends on the ability to establish and preserve differences between compartments, from the level of a single cell to the coordination of entire organs. This separation is enforced by physical boundaries built from lipids. Each boundary defines what is contained, what is excluded, and how exchange is controlled. Without these boundaries, gradients collapse, concentrations equalize, and the conditions required for organized activity disappear. The system does not begin with reactions. It begins with the ability to hold distinct internal states.

Cell membranes form the primary layer of this organization. They create a controlled interface where transport is regulated rather than allowed to occur freely. Channels, transporters, and receptors operate within this boundary, but their function depends on the stability of the structure that holds them in place. If the membrane becomes too permeable, ions move across it without control, forcing the cell to expend energy to restore separation. If it becomes too rigid, necessary exchanges slow or fail. The boundary must hold a narrow range of physical properties to maintain function. These properties are determined by the lipids that compose it, not by the energy moving through it.

This principle extends inward. Organelles maintain their own boundaries, each with specific compositions that define their role. The nucleus isolates genetic material while allowing selective transport of regulatory molecules. The mitochondrion maintains a steep gradient across its inner membrane, enabling controlled energy conversion. The endoplasmic reticulum forms a network where synthesis and processing occur within a defined environment. Each of these compartments depends on its boundary to maintain the conditions required for its function. When those boundaries degrade, the processes they support lose precision or fail entirely.

Gradients are the operational currency of the system, and gradients only exist when boundaries hold. Differences in ion concentration, electrical charge, and chemical composition drive movement and enable work to be performed. When separation is maintained, gradients can be established and used efficiently. When separation weakens, gradients dissipate, and the system shifts into constant correction. Energy is diverted toward maintaining basic differences rather than performing higher-level functions. This increases demand without improving output, creating a state where the system is active but inefficient.

At larger scales, tissues and organs rely on coordinated boundaries to function as integrated systems. Epithelial layers control what enters and exits the body. Vascular endothelium regulates exchange between blood and tissue. Neural networks depend on membrane stability to transmit signals with speed and accuracy. These structures are not independent. They operate as a continuous boundary system, where local instability can propagate into systemic effects. A disruption at the cellular level can scale into tissue dysfunction because the same structural principles apply across levels.

The body does not manage complexity by increasing reaction rates or energy throughput. It manages complexity by maintaining organized separation. Boundaries allow different processes to occur simultaneously without interference. They create controlled environments where specific reactions can proceed under defined conditions. When this organization is intact, the system operates with clarity. When it breaks down, processes overlap, signals interfere, and the distinction between compartments begins to blur.

Understanding the body as a boundary-defined system reframes how inputs are evaluated. Materials that reinforce boundary integrity support the entire system. Materials that weaken boundaries introduce instability that propagates across functions. This is not an abstract effect. It is a direct consequence of how physical structures behave under load. The body maintains order by maintaining separation, and that separation is built from lipids that determine whether the system holds or begins to lose coherence.

Lipids as the Primary Structural Material

The body is constructed from materials that determine how it holds shape, maintains separation, and supports function under load. Lipids form the core of that material system. Every cell, organelle, and transport interface depends on lipid assemblies to create boundaries that are flexible enough to allow controlled movement yet stable enough to preserve internal conditions. These assemblies are not inert layers. Their composition sets the physical properties of the system, including thickness, packing density, permeability, and electrical resistance. When lipid composition shifts, these properties shift in parallel, altering how the system behaves at every level.

Phospholipids provide the foundational framework. Their amphipathic structure drives self-assembly into bilayers, orienting hydrophilic heads outward and hydrophobic tails inward to create a continuous barrier. This arrangement determines baseline permeability. Water and small nonpolar molecules pass differently than ions and polar compounds, and the membrane enforces that distinction without constant energy input. Cholesterol intercalates within this framework and regulates packing. It limits excessive movement when membranes become too fluid and prevents tight packing when they become too rigid, maintaining a narrow operating range where transporters and receptors can function consistently. The ratio of saturated to unsaturated fatty acids further tunes this environment. Saturated chains pack tightly and resist deformation. Unsaturated chains introduce kinks that increase spacing and mobility. The balance between them determines whether the membrane holds structure under stress or drifts into instability.

These material properties control protein behavior. Membrane proteins do not function independently of their surroundings. Their orientation, movement, and interaction rates depend on the lipid environment that supports them. Receptors require specific packing conditions to cluster and initiate signaling. Transporters rely on membrane thickness and fluidity to cycle between conformations. Enzymes embedded within membranes depend on local composition to maintain catalytic efficiency. When lipid structure becomes inconsistent, protein function becomes inconsistent, even when protein levels remain unchanged. The system does not fail from a lack of components. It fails because the environment no longer supports reliable operation.

Electrical behavior is set by lipid structure as well. Ion gradients are held across membranes because the lipid bilayer resists free ion movement. This resistance allows cells to store potential and release it in controlled ways. If the membrane becomes more permeable due to altered lipid composition or oxidative damage, ions leak and gradients weaken. The cell compensates by increasing active transport, raising energy demand without improving output. Over time, this shifts the system into a state where energy is consumed maintaining separation rather than performing work. The difference between efficient and inefficient systems is not how much energy they receive, but how well their structure preserves the conditions required to use that energy.

Lipid material also determines durability under chemical stress. Double bonds within unsaturated fatty acids introduce points of vulnerability where oxidation can occur. When these sites are attacked, lipid chains break or form reactive byproducts that disrupt membrane organization. This increases permeability and distorts local signaling environments. Saturated lipids lack these reactive sites and maintain structural integrity under the same conditions. The distribution of these materials within membranes therefore sets the threshold at which damage accumulates. Systems built with more stable lipids resist disruption. Systems built with more fragile lipids require constant repair and operate closer to failure.

The body maintains this structure through continuous remodeling. Lipids are not fixed once incorporated. They are replaced over time as new materials enter through diet and existing components are removed or repaired. This process integrates incoming lipids directly into the architecture of the system. The properties of membranes gradually shift to reflect the available material pool. If that pool favors stability, membranes become more coherent and resistant to disruption. If it favors instability, those characteristics accumulate within the system. The outcome is not immediate, but it is consistent because the structure is being rebuilt continuously from the same inputs.

Recognizing lipids as the primary structural material clarifies why changes in diet produce systemic effects that extend beyond energy balance.

Lipids do not simply pass through the body. They become the body. They define the environment in which all biological processes occur. When the material is stable, processes align and operate with precision. When the material is unstable, variability emerges across systems that depend on consistent conditions. The behavior of the organism reflects the properties of the material it is built from, and those properties are determined by the lipids that form its structure.

Separation, Containment, and Controlled Exchange

Biological function depends on the ability to maintain differences. Every process requires distinct internal conditions that must be preserved against constant external pressure toward equilibrium. This is achieved through separation, enforced by lipid boundaries that hold compartments apart while permitting selective interaction. Containment is not passive. It is an active physical state where gradients are maintained, concentrations are controlled, and reactions occur within defined limits. Without this containment, chemical identity dissolves, gradients collapse, and the system loses the conditions required to produce organized output.

Membranes establish this separation by creating a barrier that restricts free movement while embedding mechanisms for controlled exchange. Ions, metabolites, and signaling molecules do not move arbitrarily across this boundary. Their passage is mediated by channels, transporters, and carriers whose behavior depends on the properties of the lipid environment. The membrane sets the baseline resistance to movement, while proteins provide regulated pathways that open, close, and cycle in response to specific conditions. This arrangement allows the system to maintain internal stability while still interacting with its surroundings in a precise and directed way.

Containment allows gradients to exist, and gradients drive function. Differences in ion concentration generate electrical potential. Differences in chemical composition create directional flow. These gradients are not static stores of energy. They are dynamic conditions that enable work to be performed when pathways are opened. If the boundary weakens, these gradients dissipate. Ions leak across membranes, concentrations equalize, and the system must expend energy to restore separation. This shifts the system from controlled operation into constant correction, increasing demand without increasing output.

Controlled exchange ensures that movement across boundaries is purposeful rather than random. Nutrients are transported into cells according to need and availability. Waste products are removed in a regulated manner. Signals are transmitted when receptors engage and pathways activate. Each of these processes depends on the integrity of the boundary. If membrane composition alters permeability, transport becomes either excessive or insufficient. If receptor environments degrade, signals are initiated or terminated incorrectly. The system continues to exchange with its environment, but the exchange loses precision, leading to accumulation of error over time.

This framework extends across all levels of organization. Cellular membranes maintain internal chemistry. Organelle membranes isolate specialized processes. Tissue barriers regulate interaction between compartments. The same principles apply at each level: separation maintains identity, containment preserves conditions, and controlled exchange enables function. Disruption at any level propagates outward because each boundary is part of a larger system of coordinated separation.

The materials that form these boundaries determine how effectively they perform these roles. Lipid composition sets permeability, resistance to stress, and susceptibility to damage. Stable structures maintain separation with minimal energy expenditure. Unstable structures require continuous correction and remain prone to failure under load. The difference is not conceptual. It is a direct consequence of how physical materials behave when subjected to chemical and electrical gradients.

Understanding separation, containment, and controlled exchange as material properties rather than abstract concepts clarifies how the system maintains order. The body does not rely on constant intervention to keep processes aligned. It relies on boundaries that hold conditions steady and allow interaction only when it is required. When those boundaries are constructed from appropriate materials, function emerges with consistency. When they are not, variability increases because the system can no longer control how it exchanges with its environment.

Why Structure Precedes All Function

Function does not arise in open space. It requires defined conditions that determine what reactions can occur, how quickly they proceed, and how their outputs are contained. Structure establishes those conditions before any function can exist. Without a boundary to hold concentration differences, substrates diffuse, gradients collapse, and reaction pathways lose direction. The cell does not begin by performing work. It begins by creating a space in which work can be performed without interference. That space is constructed from lipid membranes that enforce separation and define the environment in which all subsequent activity takes place.

Every functional process depends on constraints set by structure. Enzymatic reactions require specific concentrations of substrates and cofactors. Signal transduction depends on spatial organization, where receptors and downstream components are positioned within defined regions of the membrane. Energy production relies on the ability to maintain gradients across tightly controlled boundaries. These are not optional conditions that improve efficiency. They are prerequisites. When structure is intact, reactions proceed with predictable rates and outcomes. When structure degrades, those same reactions become inconsistent because the conditions required for their execution are no longer stable.

Membranes determine how molecules move, and movement determines interaction. Transport is not governed solely by the presence of channels or carriers. It is governed by the physical properties of the membrane that surrounds them. Permeability sets the baseline for diffusion. Thickness and fluidity influence how transport proteins change shape and cycle between states. Electrical resistance determines how well ion gradients are preserved. These structural variables define the operating range of the system. If they shift, transport behavior shifts, altering substrate availability and reaction rates across the entire network.

Signal generation and interpretation are equally dependent on structure. Receptors require organized lipid environments to cluster and initiate signaling cascades. Downstream components depend on proximity and orientation to propagate signals with precision. When membrane organization is lost, signaling becomes fragmented. Signals may initiate without proper amplification or persist beyond their intended duration due to delayed termination. The system continues to receive input, but the interpretation of that input becomes unreliable because the structural context that defines signal behavior has changed.

Energy production provides a clear example of structure setting the limits of function. The mitochondrial inner membrane maintains a proton gradient that drives ATP synthesis. This gradient exists only because the membrane restricts proton movement. If the membrane becomes permeable, protons leak, and the gradient weakens. The system compensates by increasing electron flow, which raises reactive byproduct formation and further degrades the structure. Energy continues to enter the system, but its conversion becomes inefficient because the structural conditions required for controlled conversion are compromised. Function does not fail from lack of input. It fails because structure no longer supports it.

Time reinforces the precedence of structure. Structural changes accumulate through continuous remodeling, gradually altering the conditions under which all functions operate. As membranes incorporate different lipid compositions, their properties shift, changing how transport, signaling, and energy production behave. These changes occur before measurable functional outcomes appear. By the time dysfunction is detected, the underlying structure has already moved outside its optimal range. Addressing function without correcting structure leads to temporary adjustments that do not resolve the conditions producing the problem.

Recognizing that structure precedes function aligns biological behavior with physical constraints. The system operates according to the properties of the materials that define it. When those materials support stable boundaries, functions align and produce consistent outcomes. When they do not, variability emerges across processes that depend on those boundaries. Function is not an independent layer that can be adjusted in isolation. It is the expression of the structure in which it occurs, and its reliability is determined by whether that structure can hold the conditions required for controlled operation.

Chapter 2

Membrane Architecture

Membranes are the governing structures of the biological system. They are not passive layers that separate compartments. They are engineered materials whose composition determines how the system holds gradients, transmits signals, and regulates exchange under continuously changing conditions. Every membrane operates within a narrow range of physical properties that must be maintained for the system to remain stable. These properties are set by the arrangement of lipids within the bilayer, the presence of sterols that regulate packing, and the distribution of embedded proteins that depend on that environment to function. When this architecture is coherent, the system operates with precision. When it drifts, instability emerges across every process that depends on it.

The bilayer forms through the self-assembly of phospholipids, but its behavior is not defined by that assembly alone. The fatty acid chains that make up the interior of the membrane determine how tightly the structure holds together. Saturated chains align closely, creating a dense environment that resists deformation and limits uncontrolled permeability. Unsaturated chains introduce bends that prevent tight packing, increasing fluidity and allowing movement within the membrane plane. This balance between density and mobility sets the operating range for the system. Too much rigidity restricts transport and protein function. Too much fluidity increases leakage and destabilizes gradients. The membrane must maintain a controlled midpoint where movement is possible without losing containment.

Cholesterol acts as a regulator within this system, inserting itself between phospholipids and adjusting how they interact. Its presence reduces excessive motion in fluid membranes and disrupts overly rigid packing when membranes become too dense. This stabilizing effect allows the membrane to maintain consistent behavior across temperature changes and mechanical stress. Without this regulation, membranes would fluctuate outside their functional range, leading to unpredictable transport and signaling. Cholesterol does not serve as a passive filler. It sets the boundaries within which membrane dynamics can operate.

Membrane architecture also defines how proteins behave. Embedded proteins are not independent units. Their function depends on the surrounding lipid environment. Receptors require specific packing conditions to cluster and initiate signaling. Transporters rely on membrane thickness and fluidity to cycle between conformations. Ion channels depend on local electrical properties to open and close with precision. When the lipid environment shifts, these proteins change behavior even if their structure remains unchanged. The membrane sets the context in which they operate, and any alteration to that context alters the output of the system.

Microdomains form within the membrane where specific lipids concentrate to create localized environments with distinct properties. These regions organize receptors and signaling molecules into functional clusters, allowing signals to be transmitted with speed and accuracy. The formation of these domains depends on lipid composition and the presence of stabilizing components such as cholesterol and sphingolipids. When the membrane lacks the materials required to maintain these domains, signaling becomes dispersed. Receptors no longer cluster effectively, and signals lose strength or persist beyond their intended duration. The system continues to process input, but the clarity of that processing declines.

The membrane also functions as an electrical barrier. It separates charges and allows the system to maintain gradients that drive transport and communication. The ability to hold this separation depends on the integrity of the lipid bilayer. If permeability increases due to structural instability or oxidative damage, ions cross the membrane without control. The system compensates by increasing active transport, raising energy demand while reducing efficiency. Over time, this leads to a state where energy is consumed maintaining gradients rather than performing useful work. The difference between efficient and inefficient systems is not how much energy they receive, but how well their membranes preserve the conditions required to use that energy.

Membrane architecture is continuously remodeled. Lipids are replaced as new materials enter the system, and damaged components are removed or repaired. This process integrates dietary inputs directly into the structure of the membrane. The properties of the membrane therefore reflect the composition of the available lipid pool. Stable inputs lead to membranes that resist deformation and maintain consistent behavior. Unstable inputs introduce variability, increasing susceptibility to damage and altering how the membrane responds under stress. These changes accumulate over time, gradually shifting the operating characteristics of the system.

Understanding membrane architecture provides a direct link between material input and system behavior. It explains how structural changes propagate into functional outcomes without requiring separate explanations for each process. The membrane is not one component among many. It is the medium through which all components interact. When its architecture is maintained within its functional range, processes align and produce consistent results. When it is not, variability emerges because the conditions required for coordinated activity are no longer present.

Phospholipid Bilayers as Dynamic Systems

The phospholipid bilayer is not a fixed barrier. It is a dynamic material that maintains separation while continuously adapting to mechanical, chemical, and electrical demands. Each phospholipid contains a polar head group and hydrophobic tails, which drives spontaneous organization into a bilayer that shields the tails from water while exposing the heads to it. This arrangement creates a stable interface, but stability does not mean rigidity. Individual lipids move laterally within the plane of the membrane, rotate, and adjust their packing in response to changes in composition and stress. This constant movement allows the membrane to absorb deformation, reorganize local regions, and maintain integrity without fracturing under load.

Fluidity defines how this system behaves. The degree of movement within the bilayer is controlled by the composition of the fatty acid chains. Saturated chains align closely and restrict motion, increasing resistance to deformation and limiting uncontrolled permeability. Unsaturated chains introduce bends that prevent tight packing, increasing mobility and allowing proteins embedded in the membrane to shift position and interact. The membrane operates within a narrow range where movement is sufficient to support function but constrained enough to preserve containment. If fluidity rises too far, the membrane loses its ability to hold gradients. If it drops too low, transport processes slow and protein conformational changes become restricted.

This dynamic behavior supports protein function. Membrane proteins depend on the surrounding lipid environment to maintain orientation and cycle through their functional states. Transporters require space to shift between inward-facing and outward-facing conformations. Receptors rely on lateral movement to cluster and initiate signaling. Enzymes embedded within the membrane require consistent local conditions to maintain catalytic activity. The bilayer provides both the structural support and the flexibility required for these processes to occur. When lipid composition shifts outside its functional range, protein behavior becomes inconsistent because the environment no longer supports reliable operation.

The bilayer also responds to external forces. Mechanical stress, temperature changes, and chemical exposure all influence how lipids pack and move. Cholesterol moderates these responses by inserting between phospholipids and stabilizing their interactions. When the membrane becomes too fluid, cholesterol limits excessive motion. When it becomes too rigid, cholesterol disrupts tight packing and restores mobility. This regulation allows the bilayer to maintain functional properties across varying conditions. Without it, the membrane would drift into states where either leakage or rigidity compromises system performance.

Permeability is controlled through this dynamic structure. Small nonpolar molecules can pass through the lipid interior, while ions and polar compounds require transport mechanisms. The rate at which substances cross the membrane depends on how tightly lipids are packed and how often transient spaces form between them. Increased fluidity raises the likelihood of these transient openings, increasing passive permeability. Decreased fluidity reduces these events, strengthening containment but limiting diffusion. The bilayer must balance these opposing demands to maintain controlled exchange.

The bilayer is also subject to continuous remodeling. Lipids are replaced over time as new molecules are incorporated and damaged ones are removed. This alters the distribution of saturated and unsaturated chains, changes cholesterol interactions, and shifts the overall behavior of the membrane. These changes do not occur instantly. They accumulate through repeated cycles of incorporation, gradually altering how the bilayer responds to stress and how it supports embedded proteins. The system adapts to the materials available, and the properties of the bilayer reflect the composition of that material pool.

Viewing the phospholipid bilayer as a dynamic system explains how membranes maintain both stability and adaptability. It holds separation while allowing movement. It supports protein function while regulating permeability. It absorbs stress without losing integrity. These capabilities emerge from the physical properties of the lipids themselves and how they are arranged within the membrane. When this arrangement is maintained within its functional range, the system operates with consistency. When it shifts beyond that range, variability emerges because the membrane can no longer provide the conditions required for controlled behavior.

Cholesterol as Structural Regulator, Not Risk Factor

Cholesterol functions as a control element within membrane architecture. It does not sit on the periphery of the system as a circulating liability. It is embedded within membranes where it regulates how lipids pack, how proteins behave, and how the membrane responds to stress. Its structure allows it to insert between phospholipid tails, aligning with them while interrupting excessive movement. This positioning gives cholesterol the ability to modulate membrane properties directly, adjusting fluidity, permeability, and mechanical stability in real time as conditions change.

Membranes require a narrow operating range to function correctly. If the bilayer becomes too fluid, transient gaps form more frequently, increasing passive leakage of ions and small molecules. This weakens gradients and forces the cell to expend energy restoring separation. If the bilayer becomes too rigid, transport slows and proteins embedded in the membrane struggle to shift between functional states. Cholesterol stabilizes both extremes. In highly fluid membranes, it reduces motion and tightens packing, limiting uncontrolled permeability. In overly rigid membranes, it disrupts tight alignment of saturated lipids, restoring mobility. This bidirectional control keeps the membrane within a functional range where containment and flexibility are balanced.

This regulatory role extends to protein behavior. Receptors, ion channels, and transporters depend on consistent membrane properties to maintain orientation and function. Cholesterol influences the local environment around these proteins, affecting how they cluster, how they respond to ligands, and how they cycle through conformational states. In signaling regions, cholesterol contributes to the formation of ordered domains where receptors can assemble into functional complexes. When cholesterol levels within the membrane fall outside optimal ranges, these domains lose coherence. Receptors either fail to cluster effectively or remain active longer than intended, distorting signal timing and strength.

Electrical stability also depends on cholesterol-mediated control of membrane permeability. Ion gradients are maintained because the lipid bilayer resists free movement of charged particles. When membrane structure becomes unstable, ions leak, and the cell increases active transport to compensate. Cholesterol reduces this leakage by tightening the bilayer, preserving the separation required to hold gradients with minimal energy expenditure. This directly influences how efficiently cells maintain electrical potential and how consistently they can transmit signals across tissues.

Cholesterol also affects membrane resilience under chemical stress. Lipid bilayers are exposed to reactive species that can disrupt fatty acid chains and alter membrane integrity. By stabilizing lipid packing, cholesterol reduces the susceptibility of the membrane to structural disruption. It does not prevent chemical reactions from occurring, but it limits the extent to which those reactions propagate into large-scale changes in membrane behavior. This containment preserves function under conditions that would otherwise push the system into instability.

The body maintains cholesterol distribution through tightly regulated transport systems. Lipoproteins move cholesterol between tissues, delivering it where structural reinforcement is required and removing excess when balance shifts. This process is not random circulation. It is targeted allocation of structural material. When tissues experience stress or damage, cholesterol is directed toward those regions to support repair and restore membrane integrity. Elevated levels in circulation often reflect increased demand for structural reinforcement rather than a primary cause of dysfunction.

Reframing cholesterol as a structural regulator clarifies its role within the system. It is not an external risk factor acting independently of cellular function. It is a component of the membrane that determines how the system holds its shape, maintains gradients, and supports signaling. Removing or suppressing it without addressing underlying structural conditions alters membrane behavior in ways that can reduce stability rather than improve it. The system depends on cholesterol to maintain control over its boundaries, and its presence reflects the need to keep those boundaries within a functional range where biological processes can operate with precision.

Saturation, Fluidity, and Mechanical Stability

Membrane behavior is set by how lipid chains pack together. Saturation determines that packing. Saturated fatty acids align closely, forming a dense interior that resists deformation and limits uncontrolled permeability. Unsaturated fatty acids introduce bends along the chain that prevent tight alignment, increasing spacing and lateral movement within the bilayer. This difference in geometry sets the baseline for fluidity, which then defines how the membrane responds to stress, how proteins move, and how gradients are preserved under load.

Fluidity is not a target to maximize. It is a parameter that must remain within a functional range. When the bilayer becomes too fluid, transient gaps form more frequently between lipid chains. These openings allow ions and small molecules to pass without regulation, weakening gradients and forcing the cell to increase active transport to restore separation. The system becomes energetically inefficient because it is compensating for structural leakage. When the bilayer becomes too rigid, the opposite constraint appears. Transporters and channels struggle to cycle between conformations, receptor mobility decreases, and signaling becomes delayed or incomplete. The membrane must hold a midpoint where movement is sufficient for function but constrained enough to maintain containment.

Mechanical stability emerges from this balance. A membrane built with a higher proportion of saturated lipids maintains shape under pressure, resists shear forces, and limits deformation when exposed to changes in temperature or chemical stress. This stability allows gradients to persist with minimal correction and provides a consistent environment for embedded proteins. Introducing unsaturation increases flexibility, allowing the membrane to adapt to movement and local changes in curvature, but it also reduces resistance to disruption. Each additional double bond introduces a point where packing is weakened and susceptibility to chemical attack increases. The system trades stability for mobility, and that trade must be controlled.

Cholesterol modulates this relationship by adjusting packing density in both directions. It reduces excessive motion in highly unsaturated regions and disrupts overly tight packing in saturated regions, maintaining a consistent operating range across different conditions. This regulation allows membranes to remain functional despite variations in temperature and mechanical stress. Without it, shifts in lipid composition would push the membrane outside its functional range, leading either to leakage or rigidity that interferes with protein function.

Protein behavior reflects these structural conditions. Receptors require lateral movement to cluster and initiate signaling. Transporters depend on membrane flexibility to change shape and move substrates across the bilayer. Ion channels rely on consistent electrical properties to open and close with precision. When fluidity is too high, these processes lose specificity because the environment becomes disordered. When fluidity is too low, processes slow or fail because movement is restricted. The membrane does not simply host these proteins. It defines the conditions under which they operate.

The distribution of saturated and unsaturated lipids is not static. Membranes are continuously remodeled, incorporating new lipids as they become available and replacing damaged components. Over time, this shifts the balance between rigidity and fluidity. A consistent supply of stable, saturated and monounsaturated lipids supports membranes that hold structure while maintaining controlled flexibility. A shift toward highly unsaturated inputs increases variability, raising the likelihood of leakage, oxidative damage, and signaling distortion. These changes accumulate gradually, altering how the system behaves under both normal and stressed conditions.

Mechanical stability, then, is not a fixed property. It is the result of ongoing material integration that determines how the membrane responds to force, maintains gradients, and supports protein function. When the balance between saturation and fluidity is maintained, the system operates with consistency. When it is not, the membrane becomes either too permissive or too restrictive, and the processes that depend on it begin to lose precision.

Electrical Properties of Membranes

Membranes function as electrical components that store, separate, and control charge. The lipid bilayer acts as a dielectric barrier that resists the movement of ions, allowing differences in charge to be maintained across its thickness. This separation creates membrane potential, a stored form of energy that drives transport, signaling, and coordinated activity across tissues. The ability to hold this charge is not abstract. It depends on the physical properties of the membrane, including thickness, packing density, and permeability, all of which are determined by lipid composition.

Charge separation exists because ions cannot pass freely through the hydrophobic interior of the bilayer. Instead, their movement is restricted to specific pathways provided by channels and transporters. This controlled access allows the system to build gradients and release them in a regulated manner. When channels open, ions move along these gradients, generating electrical signals or driving transport processes. When channels close, the membrane maintains separation, preserving potential for future use. This cycle depends on the membrane's ability to resist leakage. If permeability increases, ions cross without control, reducing the difference in charge and weakening the system's ability to generate signals.

Membrane composition directly influences this resistance. Tightly packed lipids increase electrical insulation by limiting the formation of transient spaces where ions could pass. Loosely packed regions increase the likelihood of leakage, reducing the stability of the gradient. Cholesterol contributes by regulating packing, maintaining a level of insulation that supports consistent electrical behavior. When lipid composition shifts toward greater instability, resistance decreases, and the membrane behaves less like a controlled barrier and more like a leaky interface. The system compensates by increasing active transport, expending energy to restore gradients that no longer hold passively.

Electrical properties are not confined to isolated cells. They scale across tissues and systems. Neurons rely on rapid changes in membrane potential to transmit signals along axons. Muscle cells depend on controlled depolarization to initiate contraction. Epithelial tissues use electrical gradients to regulate transport across barriers. In each case, the speed, strength, and precision of these processes depend on the integrity of the membrane that holds the underlying charge. Variations in membrane composition alter how quickly potentials can be generated and how long they can be maintained, affecting the performance of entire systems.

Capacitance, the ability of the membrane to store charge, also depends on structure. The thickness of the bilayer and the arrangement of its components determine how much charge can be held for a given difference in potential. A stable membrane with consistent composition maintains predictable capacitance, allowing signals to propagate with defined timing. Structural inconsistency alters this property, introducing variability in how signals are initiated and transmitted. The result is not simply weaker signals, but less reliable timing, where activation and recovery phases begin to overlap or drift.

Ion channels and transporters operate within this electrical framework. Their opening and closing depend on changes in voltage, ligand binding, or mechanical forces, but their behavior is influenced by the membrane environment. Changes in lipid composition alter how these proteins respond to stimuli, shifting thresholds for activation and affecting the duration of open states. This modifies how ions flow and how electrical signals are shaped. The system continues to function, but the precision of that function declines as structural conditions move outside their optimal range.

Electrical stability requires that gradients be maintained with minimal correction. When membranes hold charge effectively, energy can be directed toward productive work such as signal transmission and coordinated contraction. When membranes leak, energy is diverted toward restoring gradients, increasing baseline demand without improving output. Over time, this shifts the system into a state where electrical processes remain active but operate with reduced efficiency and increased variability.

Understanding membranes as electrical structures clarifies how changes in lipid composition translate into changes in system behavior. The membrane is not simply a boundary. It is the medium through which electrical energy is stored and controlled. Its ability to maintain charge determines how signals are generated, how they propagate, and how reliably they terminate. When this structure is stable, electrical processes operate with precision. When it is not, variability emerges because the system can no longer maintain the conditions required for controlled charge separation.

Chapter 3

Lipid Organization and Microdomains

Membranes do not operate as uniform sheets of lipid. Their function depends on internal organization, where specific lipids cluster to form regions with distinct physical properties. These regions, often referred to as microdomains, create localized environments that control how proteins interact, how signals initiate, and how information moves across the membrane. Without this organization, signaling components would be dispersed across the membrane surface, reducing the probability of interaction and weakening the system's ability to produce coordinated responses. The membrane is not simply a boundary. It is a structured platform that arranges functional elements into operational units.

Microdomain formation arises from differences in lipid composition. Certain lipids, particularly those with saturated chains and higher affinity for cholesterol, pack more tightly and form ordered regions within the bilayer. These regions coexist with less ordered areas composed of more fluid lipids. The contrast between these environments creates spatial separation within the membrane, allowing specific proteins to localize where conditions support their function. Receptors, signaling complexes, and transport systems concentrate within these domains, increasing interaction rates and ensuring that signals are processed with speed and accuracy.

This organization determines how signals are initiated. Receptors often require clustering to activate downstream pathways. When localized within a microdomain, they are positioned in close proximity, allowing ligand binding to trigger coordinated activation rather than isolated responses. The membrane provides the structural context that enables this clustering. If lipid composition supports domain formation, signaling becomes efficient and controlled. If that composition shifts and domains lose coherence, receptors disperse. Activation becomes inconsistent, requiring higher input to produce the same response or generating signals that fail to propagate effectively.

Signal amplification depends on this spatial arrangement. Once receptors are activated, downstream components must interact in sequence. Microdomains bring these components into proximity, reducing the time required for interaction and limiting signal loss. The membrane effectively creates a confined environment where signaling molecules can move and interact without interference from unrelated processes. When this organization degrades, signaling pathways become fragmented. Components that should interact remain separated, slowing transmission and increasing variability in output.

Termination of signaling also relies on membrane organization. Signals must be shut down once their function is complete to prevent continuous activation. Enzymes responsible for deactivating signals are often localized within or near the same domains where activation occurs. This proximity ensures that once a signal has been transmitted, it can be rapidly terminated. If domain structure is lost, termination becomes delayed or incomplete, leading to prolonged activation and accumulation of overlapping signals. The system shifts from precise control to persistent noise, where multiple pathways remain active without clear resolution.

Microdomains influence not only signaling but also transport and structural integrity. Ion channels and transporters often localize within these regions, where the surrounding lipid environment supports their function. The mechanical properties of the domain determine how these proteins respond to stimuli and how efficiently they move substrates across the membrane. Changes in domain composition alter these properties, affecting transport rates and the ability to maintain gradients. The membrane does not simply host these processes. It organizes them into functional zones that determine their behavior.

The stability of microdomains depends on the availability of specific lipids and the presence of cholesterol to regulate packing. When the lipid pool shifts toward compositions that do not support ordered regions, domain formation becomes unstable. This does not eliminate signaling or transport, but it reduces their precision. Processes that once operated within defined environments begin to overlap, increasing interference and reducing clarity. The system continues to function, but with increased variability and reduced efficiency.

Continuous remodeling of membranes integrates new lipids into this organizational framework. Over time, the composition of microdomains shifts based on the materials available. Stable inputs support the formation of coherent domains that maintain consistent signaling environments. Unstable inputs introduce variability, making domains less defined and more susceptible to disruption. These changes accumulate, altering how the system processes information and responds to input.

Lipid organization at the level of microdomains provides the structural basis for coordinated function. It explains how membranes support complex signaling without requiring centralized control. By arranging components into localized environments, the membrane enables rapid, precise interaction while maintaining separation between unrelated processes. When this organization is intact, signaling is clear and controlled. When it is not, the system loses coherence because the structural framework required for coordination is no longer present.

Lipid Rafts and Signal Localization

Signal transmission at the membrane is not governed by random encounters. It depends on spatial concentration, where receptors and their associated machinery are positioned within defined regions that support rapid interaction. Lipid rafts provide this structure. They are localized domains enriched in cholesterol, sphingolipids, and more saturated lipid species that pack into a tighter, more ordered arrangement than the surrounding membrane. This ordered state creates a distinct physical environment where specific proteins preferentially localize, allowing signaling components to assemble into functional units rather than remaining dispersed across the membrane surface.

The formation of these domains is driven by lipid compatibility. Saturated chains align with cholesterol to create regions of reduced fluidity and increased packing density. This environment excludes lipids that do not fit this arrangement, leading to phase separation within the membrane. The result is a mosaic structure where ordered and less ordered regions coexist. Proteins with affinity for these ordered domains concentrate within them, creating zones where receptors, co-receptors, and downstream signaling elements are positioned in close proximity. This proximity reduces the time required for interaction and increases the probability that a signal will propagate effectively once initiated.

Localization within lipid rafts alters how signals are initiated. Receptors often require clustering to transition from an inactive to an active state. Within a raft, the density of compatible lipids and associated proteins supports this clustering. Ligand binding to one receptor increases the likelihood that neighboring receptors will also engage, producing a coordinated activation rather than isolated events. This changes the strength and clarity of the signal at its point of origin. Outside of these domains, receptors are more dispersed, and activation events are less likely to propagate, leading to weaker or inconsistent signaling.

Signal amplification depends on maintaining this localized environment. Once receptors activate, downstream molecules must interact in sequence to transmit the signal. Lipid rafts act as confined spaces where these interactions occur with minimal interference from unrelated processes. The ordered environment stabilizes protein interactions and supports the formation of signaling complexes that persist long enough to complete their function. When these domains are intact, signaling proceeds with defined timing and strength. When they are disrupted, components disperse, and interactions become less efficient, reducing the ability of the system to amplify input into a coherent response.

Termination of signaling is also influenced by raft integrity. Enzymes responsible for deactivating signaling molecules often localize within or near these domains, allowing rapid shutdown once a signal has been transmitted. This spatial arrangement ensures that activation and termination occur within the same controlled environment. If raft structure is lost, termination becomes less coordinated. Signals persist beyond their intended duration, leading to overlapping activation states that increase noise within the system.

The physical properties of lipid rafts also affect how the membrane responds to mechanical and electrical stress. Their tighter packing increases local resistance to deformation and reduces permeability, helping maintain gradients and stabilize electrical potential. Proteins embedded within these domains operate under more consistent conditions, which supports predictable behavior. Changes in lipid composition that weaken raft formation reduce this stability, making signaling and transport more susceptible to disruption under load.

Raft stability depends on the availability of cholesterol and compatible lipid species. When these components are present in appropriate proportions, domains form and persist long enough to support organized signaling. When the balance shifts toward lipids that do not support ordered packing, these domains fragment or fail to form. The system does not stop signaling, but the organization required for precision is lost. Receptors become dispersed, interactions slow, and signals degrade in strength and timing.

Continuous membrane remodeling integrates new lipids into this system, gradually altering the distribution and stability of rafts. Stable inputs support the maintenance of ordered domains, reinforcing consistent signaling environments. Inputs that disrupt packing introduce variability, reducing the coherence of these regions. Over time, this changes how signals are generated and processed across the entire system.

Lipid rafts provide the structural basis for signal localization. They ensure that signaling components are positioned where they can interact efficiently, allowing the system to convert input into coordinated output. When these domains are intact, signaling is precise and controlled. When they are not, the same inputs produce weaker, less reliable responses because the structural framework that supports localization has been compromised.

Receptor Clustering and Signal Amplification

Signal initiation at the membrane depends on density and proximity. A single receptor binding event rarely produces a meaningful output on its own. The system requires multiple receptors to engage in a coordinated manner so that downstream pathways receive a signal strong enough to propagate. Clustering provides this coordination. When receptors are positioned within defined regions of the membrane, the probability that they will interact increases, allowing individual activation events to combine into a unified signal. Without clustering, receptors remain dispersed, and activation remains isolated, reducing the likelihood that a signal will reach the threshold required for amplification.

The membrane sets the conditions for this process. Lipid composition determines whether receptors can move laterally and assemble into functional groups. In environments where packing supports controlled mobility, receptors are able to diffuse within the membrane plane and encounter one another. Once a ligand binds, it alters the conformation of the receptor, increasing its affinity for neighboring receptors and associated signaling proteins. This initiates the formation of clusters that stabilize the active state. The membrane does not simply host this interaction. It determines whether it can occur efficiently by controlling how freely receptors can move and how closely they can align.

Clustering changes the nature of the signal. Instead of a linear response to a single activation event, the system produces a nonlinear output where multiple receptors contribute simultaneously. This increases the strength of the signal and reduces the impact of random fluctuations. The system filters noise by requiring coordinated activation before downstream pathways are engaged. Once a cluster forms, signaling components are recruited to the same location, allowing rapid transmission through the pathway. The signal becomes both stronger and more reliable because it originates from a localized and coordinated source.

Signal amplification depends on maintaining this localized structure long enough for downstream interactions to occur. Proteins involved in signal transduction must bind, activate, and pass the signal along in sequence. Clusters provide a confined environment where these interactions can proceed without interruption. The density of components within the cluster increases interaction rates, reducing delays and preventing signal loss. If clustering is unstable, components disperse before the signal can fully propagate, resulting in incomplete or weakened output.

Termination of the signal also relies on the integrity of the cluster. Once the signal has been transmitted, receptors must return to their inactive state, and associated proteins must disengage. This requires coordinated disassembly of the cluster. If the membrane environment supports controlled clustering, it also supports controlled dissociation. When this balance is lost, clusters may persist longer than intended or fail to form properly. Persistent clusters lead to prolonged signaling, while incomplete clusters lead to weak or inconsistent activation. Both outcomes reflect a breakdown in the structural conditions required for precise control.

Membrane composition influences every stage of this process. Lipids that support stable packing and domain formation allow receptors to cluster efficiently and maintain coherence during activation. Lipids that introduce excessive fluidity or instability reduce the ability of receptors to remain localized, increasing dispersion and lowering the probability of effective clustering. These changes do not eliminate signaling. They alter its quality, shifting the system from coordinated amplification to fragmented responses.

Clustering also affects how the system responds to varying levels of input. In a well-organized membrane, small increases in ligand concentration can produce significant changes in output because clusters form more readily as receptor engagement increases. This creates a responsive system capable of scaling output based on input strength. When clustering is impaired, this responsiveness declines. Larger inputs are required to produce the same level of activation, and the system becomes less sensitive to changes in its environment.

Receptor clustering and signal amplification are therefore not purely biochemical events. They are structural processes governed by the physical properties of the membrane. The ability to convert input into a meaningful signal depends on whether receptors can assemble into functional groups, maintain that assembly long enough to propagate the signal, and then disassemble in a controlled manner. When the membrane supports these conditions, signaling is precise and efficient. When it does not, amplification becomes inconsistent, and the system loses its ability to respond reliably to input.

Domain Instability and Signaling Noise

Membrane domains only function when they hold their structure long enough to organize interactions. When the lipid environment no longer supports that organization, domains fragment, merge unpredictably, or fail to form at all. This instability changes how signaling components are positioned relative to one another. Receptors drift out of alignment, scaffolding proteins lose their anchoring context, and enzymes that should be co-localized become separated. The system continues to receive input, but the spatial framework that converts input into coordinated output is no longer reliable.

Fragmentation reduces local density. Signals that depend on receptor proximity fail to reach threshold because activation events remain isolated instead of combining into a unified response. At the same time, transient collisions between components increase. Proteins that would not normally interact encounter one another due to loss of spatial segregation, initiating pathways that are either weak or inappropriate for the context. The membrane becomes permissive to random interaction rather than selective interaction. This is the origin of signaling noise, where activation occurs without clear direction or fails to propagate despite adequate input.

Temporal control degrades alongside spatial control. In stable domains, activation and termination occur within the same localized environment, allowing signals to begin and end with defined timing. When domains are unstable, initiation may occur in one region while termination mechanisms are displaced or delayed. This creates overlap between signaling events. Pathways remain active longer than intended, or they terminate prematurely before completing their sequence. The system shifts from discrete signals to continuous fluctuation, where activation states blur together and lose distinction.

Electrical and chemical conditions amplify this instability. Increased membrane permeability alters local ion concentrations, affecting how voltage-sensitive components respond. Reactive byproducts generated under stress modify lipid structure, further disrupting packing and accelerating domain breakdown. These changes feed back into the system, increasing variability in both signal strength and duration. The membrane no longer provides a stable platform. It becomes a fluctuating environment where conditions change faster than signaling pathways can adapt.

Signal amplification becomes unreliable under these conditions. Clusters form inconsistently and dissolve before downstream interactions are completed. Some signals fail to propagate, while others extend beyond their intended range. The system alternates between under-response and over-response, depending on local conditions within the membrane. This variability is not random. It reflects the absence of a stable structure to constrain and guide signaling behavior.

Transport processes are affected in parallel. Channels and carriers that depend on domain organization lose their positional stability, altering how substrates move across the membrane. Gradients become harder to maintain as localized permeability changes, increasing the need for compensatory activity. Energy is diverted toward restoring baseline conditions rather than supporting coordinated function. This raises demand while reducing the efficiency of signal processing.

Domain instability does not eliminate signaling. It removes precision. The system continues to operate, but with reduced coherence, where inputs no longer produce consistent outputs. Over time, this leads to accumulation of error as pathways activate without proper context or fail to terminate cleanly. The membrane becomes a source of variability rather than a platform for control.

Restoring domain stability requires restoring the material conditions that support organized lipid packing. When membranes regain the ability to form coherent domains, signaling components realign, interaction rates normalize, and timing becomes consistent again. The system does not need additional complexity to correct noise. It requires the structural framework that allows signals to be generated, amplified, and terminated within defined boundaries.

Structural Control of Cellular Communication

Cellular communication is constrained by where components are placed and how long they remain in proximity. Signals do not travel through an empty medium. They are generated, shaped, and terminated within membranes whose composition determines interaction rates, directionality, and timing. The membrane sets encounter frequency by controlling lateral mobility, sets selectivity by organizing domains, and sets duration by governing how quickly complexes assemble and disassemble. Change the structure and the same ligands, receptors, and pathways produce different outputs because the physical context that defines their behavior has shifted.

Spatial organization defines who can interact with whom. Lipid domains concentrate compatible proteins into regions where binding and downstream activation occur with high probability. Receptors, co-receptors, kinases, and scaffolds are brought into alignment so that a binding event propagates through a defined sequence rather than diffusing across unrelated components. When this organization holds, signaling is directed. When it degrades, components disperse, and interactions become opportunistic. Activation may occur without proper partners present, or partners may fail to meet in time, producing weak or incomplete transmission.

Mobility sets the pace of communication. Lipid composition determines how freely proteins move within the membrane plane. Adequate mobility allows receptors to cluster and recruit downstream machinery. Excessive mobility prevents stable assembly, causing complexes to dissolve before signals propagate. Insufficient mobility traps components, slowing response and reducing sensitivity to changing input. The membrane therefore defines a window where movement supports assembly without compromising stability. Within this window, signals initiate and propagate with predictable timing.

Thresholding emerges from density and confinement. Local concentration within domains lowers the amount of input required to trigger a response because multiple receptors engage in a coordinated manner. This creates nonlinear behavior where small changes in ligand availability can produce large changes in output. When domains are unstable and density drops, thresholds rise. Larger inputs are required to achieve the same activation, and responses become inconsistent. The system appears less responsive not because receptors are absent, but because the structure no longer supports coordinated engagement.

Directionality depends on how pathways are arranged relative to one another. Membrane architecture places sequential components within reach so that signals move along preferred routes. Scaffolding proteins anchor elements of a pathway in defined positions, limiting cross-talk with unrelated processes. When this arrangement is disrupted, signals leak into adjacent pathways or stall due to loss of alignment. The result is overlap between responses that should remain separate, increasing interference and reducing specificity.

Timing is set by assembly and disassembly kinetics within the membrane environment. Activation requires formation of complexes that persist long enough to transmit the signal. Termination requires those complexes to break apart and for deactivating enzymes to access their targets. Membrane structure controls both processes by influencing how tightly components pack and how easily they separate. Stable domains support rapid assembly followed by controlled dissociation. Disordered membranes produce delayed assembly and prolonged persistence, leading to signals that start late and end late, overlapping with subsequent inputs.

Electrical conditions feed into this control. The membrane's ability to hold charge affects voltage-sensitive channels and receptors, altering how signals initiate and propagate. Increased permeability introduces variability in local potential, shifting activation thresholds and changing the shape of the response. Chemical conditions follow the same pattern. Oxidative changes in lipid composition alter packing and domain stability, feeding back into spatial organization and timing. Communication reflects the state of the membrane because the membrane defines the medium through which communication occurs.

At the system level, these local effects scale into coordinated behavior or widespread noise. Tissues rely on consistent signaling across many cells. When membrane structure is coherent, signals propagate with uniform timing and strength, allowing synchronization. When structure varies, cells respond differently to the same input, fragmenting the response across the tissue. The difference is not in the signal itself, but in the structural conditions that determine how that signal is processed.

Structural control reframes communication as a property of material organization rather than a sequence of isolated reactions. Inputs, receptors, and pathways remain the same, but their behavior is governed by how they are arranged and constrained within the membrane. Restore the structure and communication aligns without additional intervention. Allow the structure to drift and communication becomes variable because the system no longer enforces the conditions required for precise interaction.

Chapter 4

Mitochondrial Membranes and Energy Control

Energy production is not defined by substrate availability. It is defined by whether the mitochondrial membranes can hold and control a gradient. The mitochondrion operates as a compartment within a compartment, with an outer membrane that sets access and an inner membrane that performs the core work. The inner membrane establishes separation between matrix and intermembrane space and maintains a steep proton gradient that drives ATP synthesis. This gradient is a physical condition, not a concept. It exists only if the membrane resists proton movement and preserves charge separation under continuous flux. When that resistance holds, energy conversion proceeds with control. When it does not, the same inputs produce unstable output because the gradient cannot be maintained.

The inner membrane is specialized for this task. Its surface area is expanded through cristae, increasing the space available for the electron transport chain and ATP synthase. Proteins embedded in this membrane move electrons through a sequence of redox reactions that pump protons outward, building the gradient. The membrane must remain sufficiently impermeable to prevent those protons from returning except through ATP synthase. This constraint allows the system to couple electron flow to ATP production. If protons leak back across the membrane through uncontrolled pathways, the coupling weakens. Electron flow increases to compensate, but ATP yield per unit input declines, and reactive byproducts rise as electrons escape the chain.

Lipid composition determines whether this membrane can perform its function. Cardiolipin, a phospholipid unique to the inner mitochondrial membrane, plays a central role in stabilizing protein complexes and maintaining membrane curvature. Its structure supports tight packing and creates an environment that holds the electron transport components in close proximity. This organization reduces the distance electrons must travel and limits the opportunity for leakage. When cardiolipin is intact, the system maintains efficient electron transfer and stable gradient formation. When it is damaged or depleted, complexes lose alignment, electron flow becomes less controlled, and the membrane becomes more permeable to protons.

Permeability is the central variable in energy control. A membrane that holds protons tightly allows the gradient to build with minimal loss, enabling efficient ATP production. A membrane that allows even small increases in proton leakage shifts the system into a different operating mode. The cell compensates by increasing substrate oxidation to maintain ATP levels, raising oxygen consumption and reactive species generation. This creates a feedback loop where structural damage leads to increased stress, which further degrades the membrane. Energy is still being produced, but it is produced under conditions that reduce efficiency and increase instability.

Electrical potential across the inner membrane reflects its structural integrity. The difference in charge between the matrix and intermembrane space stores energy that can be released through ATP synthase or dissipated through leakage. Stable membranes maintain this potential within a defined range, allowing consistent control of energy output. When membrane composition shifts, the potential fluctuates. Channels and carriers respond to these changes, altering ion movement and further affecting gradient stability. The system becomes less predictable because the underlying structure no longer enforces consistent electrical conditions.

Transport into and out of the mitochondrion is also governed by membrane properties. Substrates must cross the outer membrane through channels and the inner membrane through specific transporters. These processes depend on membrane fluidity, thickness, and organization. If the membrane becomes too rigid, transport slows, limiting substrate availability. If it becomes too permeable, gradients that drive transport dissipate, reducing efficiency. The balance between containment and movement defines how effectively substrates are delivered to the sites of energy production.

Mitochondrial membranes are continuously remodeled. Lipids are replaced and repaired as the system integrates new materials. This process determines whether the membrane moves toward stability or instability over time. Inputs that support tight packing and resistance to oxidative damage reinforce the ability to maintain gradients. Inputs that introduce structural fragility increase susceptibility to leakage and degradation. The system reflects these changes gradually, altering energy production capacity before overt dysfunction appears.

Energy output, then, is not a direct function of how much fuel is available. It is constrained by how well the mitochondrial membranes hold the conditions required for controlled conversion. When structure is intact, the system produces consistent ATP with minimal waste. When structure is compromised, the system compensates by increasing throughput, but this comes at the cost of efficiency and stability. Understanding energy control requires focusing on the membrane that defines the gradient, because the gradient is the mechanism through which energy is converted into usable form.

Inner Membrane Structure and Gradient Containment

The inner mitochondrial membrane exists to hold a gradient under continuous load. Its geometry, composition, and protein density are arranged to resist proton movement while allowing controlled return through ATP synthase. Cristae fold the membrane into tightly curved compartments that increase surface area and create microenvironments where protons accumulate. These folds are not decorative. They reduce diffusion distance, concentrate charge, and place electron transport complexes and ATP synthase within defined regions so that proton flow can be captured before it dissipates. When cristae structure is intact, the gradient is locally steep and globally stable, allowing consistent energy conversion.

Containment depends on lipid packing. Cardiolipin anchors the inner membrane by supporting tight alignment of acyl chains and stabilizing curvature at the cristae. This lipid binds directly to respiratory complexes, maintaining their position and preserving the spacing required for efficient electron transfer. Dense packing reduces free volume within the bilayer, limiting passive proton movement. The membrane behaves as a barrier with selective permeability, where protons are forced to follow defined pathways. When cardiolipin is altered or oxidized, packing loosens, curvature becomes unstable, and proteins drift from their optimal positions. The barrier weakens, and protons begin to bypass ATP synthase through uncontrolled routes.

Protein organization reinforces this containment. Complexes I through IV form supercomplexes that align electron flow with proton pumping, reducing the distance between sequential steps. ATP synthase dimers localize along the ridges of cristae, positioned where the gradient is strongest. This arrangement ensures that the return of protons is captured efficiently. If these structures disperse, electron flow continues, but proton pumping becomes less coordinated. The gradient spreads across a broader area with lower intensity, and ATP synthase operates under reduced driving force. The system compensates by increasing throughput, but the coupling between oxidation and phosphorylation weakens.

Permeability is controlled at multiple levels. The lipid matrix sets baseline resistance, while embedded proteins regulate specific transport. Under stable conditions, proton leakage is minimal, and the gradient is maintained with modest electron flow. Small increases in permeability shift the operating point. Electron transport accelerates to sustain the gradient, raising oxygen consumption and increasing the probability of electron escape from the chain. This produces reactive species that further modify lipids and proteins, increasing permeability again. The cycle reinforces itself until the membrane either stabilizes through repair or continues toward greater inefficiency.

Electrical potential across the inner membrane is a direct readout of containment. A high and steady potential indicates that protons are being held and released through controlled channels. Fluctuating or reduced potential reflects leakage or disrupted organization. Ion transporters respond to these changes, adjusting fluxes of calcium and other ions that influence mitochondrial activity. When the membrane cannot maintain a stable potential, these adjustments become erratic, altering enzyme activity and further destabilizing energy production.

Gradient containment also depends on the integrity of junctions between cristae and the inner boundary membrane. These junctions restrict diffusion, allowing protons to remain concentrated within cristae rather than equilibrating across the entire intermembrane space. Structural proteins maintain these junctions. If they weaken, the gradient disperses, lowering local proton density and reducing the efficiency of ATP synthesis. The system does not stop producing energy, but it requires more input to achieve the same output because the gradient is less focused.

Maintenance of this structure requires continuous lipid turnover and repair. Damaged lipids are replaced, and new lipids are integrated into the membrane, altering its properties over time. When the balance favors stable packing and resistance to oxidative modification, containment improves. When damage accumulates faster than repair, permeability rises, and the gradient becomes harder to sustain. These changes occur gradually, shifting the operating conditions of the mitochondrion before overt failure is observed.

The inner membrane defines the boundary that makes energy conversion possible. Its ability to contain a gradient determines whether electron flow is translated into ATP or lost as heat and reactive byproducts. When the structure holds, the system operates with precision. When it does not, the same biochemical machinery produces a different outcome because the physical conditions required for controlled energy conversion are no longer enforced.

Cardiolipin and Electron Transport Chain Stability

Cardiolipin defines the operating conditions of the inner mitochondrial membrane by stabilizing both its structure and the protein complexes embedded within it. Its four acyl chains allow tighter packing than standard phospholipids, creating regions of reduced permeability and increased curvature that support cristae formation. This lipid is not distributed uniformly. It concentrates in areas where the electron transport chain is active, binding directly to complexes and holding them in position. Without this anchoring, the membrane becomes a less organized surface where proteins drift, spacing increases, and the sequence of electron transfer loses alignment.

The electron transport chain depends on proximity. Electrons move through a series of carriers that must remain within defined distances to minimize loss. Cardiolipin supports the formation of supercomplexes, where multiple respiratory complexes assemble into stable units. This arrangement reduces the diffusion distance for electron carriers such as coenzyme Q and cytochrome c, allowing electrons to pass rapidly and with minimal leakage. When cardiolipin is intact, these supercomplexes remain stable, and electron flow proceeds in a controlled manner. When cardiolipin is altered, these assemblies disintegrate, increasing the distance between components and raising the probability that electrons will escape the chain.

Electron leakage changes the system's behavior. Escaped electrons react with oxygen to form reactive species that modify nearby lipids and proteins. Cardiolipin itself becomes a target, and its oxidation further weakens membrane structure. This creates a feedback loop where structural damage increases electron leakage, which then accelerates additional damage. The electron transport chain continues to operate, but it does so with reduced efficiency and increased byproduct formation. Energy production becomes coupled with rising oxidative stress because the structural conditions that limit leakage are no longer intact.

Cardiolipin also influences the activity of individual complexes. Its interaction with protein surfaces affects conformation and stability, ensuring that complexes maintain the shapes required for efficient electron transfer and proton pumping. Changes in cardiolipin composition alter these interactions. If the lipid environment no longer supports proper folding or positioning, complexes may remain present but operate less effectively. Proton pumping becomes inconsistent, weakening the gradient that drives ATP synthesis. The system compensates by increasing electron flow, but this raises substrate demand and further stresses the membrane.

Membrane curvature depends on cardiolipin distribution. The inner mitochondrial membrane is not flat. Its folds create localized environments where the gradient is concentrated and where ATP synthase operates under optimal conditions. Cardiolipin supports this curvature by stabilizing regions of high bending. When its levels decline or its structure is modified, these regions lose definition. Cristae become less organized, and the spatial relationship between electron transport complexes and ATP synthase shifts. This reduces the efficiency with which the gradient is captured and converted into ATP.

Turnover and remodeling of cardiolipin determine long-term stability. The lipid is continuously synthesized and repaired, incorporating new acyl chains and replacing damaged molecules. The composition of these chains affects how well cardiolipin can support tight packing and protein interaction. Stable compositions reinforce membrane integrity and supercomplex formation. Altered compositions introduce variability, making the membrane more susceptible to disruption under stress. Over time, these changes influence how consistently the electron transport chain can operate.

Cardiolipin therefore acts as a structural mediator between the membrane and the respiratory machinery. It holds complexes in position, maintains the curvature required for gradient concentration, and limits electron loss by preserving proximity and alignment. When its structure is maintained, electron transport proceeds with control and efficiency. When it is compromised, the same biochemical components operate in a less organized environment, leading to reduced ATP output and increased reactive byproducts because the membrane no longer enforces the conditions required for stable electron flow.

Proton Leakage and Energy Inefficiency

The inner mitochondrial membrane only produces controlled energy when protons are forced to return through ATP synthase. Any alternative pathway that allows protons to cross the membrane without passing through this enzyme breaks the coupling between electron transport and ATP production. Proton leakage is therefore not a minor side effect. It changes the operating mode of the entire system by reducing how much of the gradient can be converted into usable energy.

Leakage begins at the level of the lipid matrix. Tight packing of lipids limits the formation of transient spaces within the membrane where protons can move. When packing loosens, these spaces appear more frequently, creating routes for protons to slip across the bilayer. Even small increases in permeability have measurable effects because the gradient depends on maintaining a large difference in proton concentration across a very thin barrier. A slight increase in proton return outside ATP synthase reduces the driving force available for ATP production and lowers efficiency at every cycle of the system.

Protein-mediated pathways add another layer to this process. Uncoupling proteins and damaged channels can provide controlled or uncontrolled routes for proton movement. Under certain conditions, controlled leakage serves a function by dissipating excess gradient and limiting the buildup of reactive intermediates. Outside of those conditions, increased activity of these pathways diverts protons away from ATP synthase, forcing the system to oxidize more substrate to maintain ATP levels. The mitochondrion compensates by increasing electron transport activity, but this raises oxygen consumption and increases the likelihood of electron escape from the chain.

Electron escape amplifies the problem. As more electrons leak, reactive species form and interact with membrane lipids, altering their structure and further increasing permeability. This establishes a feedback loop where leakage drives oxidative modification, which then accelerates additional leakage. The membrane gradually loses its ability to act as a tight barrier, and the gradient becomes harder to sustain despite increased metabolic input.

Electrical potential reflects this shift. A stable membrane maintains a high potential difference, indicating that protons are being held and released through controlled pathways. As leakage increases, this potential declines or fluctuates because protons no longer remain confined. Ion transporters respond to these changes, adjusting fluxes of other ions such as calcium, which in turn affects mitochondrial activity. These adjustments introduce additional variability into the system, further reducing the predictability of energy production.

Energy inefficiency emerges from this altered state. More fuel is required to produce the same amount of ATP because a portion of the gradient is continuously lost. The system increases throughput to compensate, but this increases heat generation and reactive byproduct formation. The cell maintains ATP levels, but it does so with higher input and lower yield. Over time, this places a sustained demand on substrate supply and increases stress on the membrane, reinforcing the conditions that allow leakage to persist.

Transport processes are also affected. Many carriers rely on the gradient as a driving force to move substrates into the mitochondrion. As the gradient weakens, these processes become less effective, limiting the availability of key molecules required for energy production. The system attempts to compensate through alternative pathways, but these are less efficient and often increase metabolic burden.

Proton leakage does not stop energy production. It changes how energy is produced by shifting the system from a tightly coupled state to a partially uncoupled one. In this state, electron transport continues at an elevated rate, but a smaller fraction of the energy captured from substrate oxidation is converted into ATP. The difference is lost as heat and reactive intermediates because the membrane no longer enforces the constraint that protons must pass through ATP synthase. Restoring efficiency requires restoring the structural conditions that limit uncontrolled proton movement, because containment of the gradient is what allows the system to convert input into controlled output.

Structural Control of ATP Production

ATP production is determined by whether the inner mitochondrial membrane can impose constraint on proton movement and maintain alignment between proton flow and ATP synthase. The enzyme itself does not create energy. It converts an existing gradient into chemical work. That conversion only occurs if protons are forced to return through the enzyme rather than diffusing across the membrane. The structure of the membrane sets this condition by limiting permeability, organizing protein complexes, and maintaining the geometry required for efficient capture of the gradient. When these conditions hold, ATP output follows the gradient closely. When they do not, the same electron flow produces less ATP because the gradient is partially dissipated before it can be used.

The position of ATP synthase within the membrane is not random. Dimers of the enzyme localize along the curved edges of cristae, where proton density is highest. This placement increases the probability that returning protons will pass through the enzyme. The curvature itself is supported by lipid composition, particularly cardiolipin, which stabilizes both the shape of the membrane and the positioning of protein complexes. This creates a spatial relationship where electron transport complexes pump protons into regions that feed directly into ATP synthase. Disruption of this arrangement spreads the gradient over a larger area with lower local intensity, reducing the driving force available to each enzyme.

Coupling between electron transport and ATP synthesis depends on proximity and timing. Protons are pumped into the intermembrane space as electrons move through the chain. If ATP synthase is positioned to capture those protons immediately, the system operates efficiently. If the membrane structure allows protons to diffuse away from these sites, the effective gradient at the enzyme decreases. The system compensates by increasing electron flow, but this increases oxygen consumption and raises the probability of electron leakage. ATP production continues, but at a higher metabolic cost and with increased instability.

Membrane permeability sets the upper limit of efficiency. A tightly packed bilayer forces protons to follow defined pathways, maintaining a high electrochemical gradient. Small increases in permeability reduce this gradient even if proton pumping remains unchanged. ATP synthase responds to the reduced driving force by producing less ATP per unit time. The cell maintains energy levels by increasing substrate oxidation, but this shifts the system toward higher throughput with lower yield. The difference is released as heat and reactive byproducts because the membrane no longer enforces strict coupling.

Electrical potential integrates these effects. The voltage across the inner membrane reflects how well protons are contained and how effectively their movement is being harnessed. Stable potential supports consistent rotation of ATP synthase and steady ATP output. Fluctuating potential introduces variability in enzyme activity, leading to inconsistent production rates. Ion movements that respond to these fluctuations further influence mitochondrial conditions, reinforcing or disrupting the system depending on the direction of change.

Substrate delivery and product removal depend on the same structural conditions. Transporters embedded in the membrane rely on gradients and membrane organization to move ADP into the matrix and export ATP to the cytosol. If the gradient weakens or membrane organization shifts, these transport processes slow or become less efficient. This creates a secondary limitation where ATP production is constrained not only by synthesis but also by the movement of substrates and products across the membrane.

ATP production is therefore a structural outcome. The enzyme, substrates, and electron transport chain are necessary components, but they do not determine efficiency on their own. The membrane defines how these components interact by controlling proximity, permeability, and gradient containment. When the structure is intact, the system converts input into ATP with minimal loss. When it is compromised, the same components operate under altered conditions, producing less ATP and generating more byproducts because the physical framework required for controlled energy conversion is no longer maintained.

PART II

LIPIDS AS SIGNALING INFRASTRUCTURE

Chapter 5

Lipids as Information Carriers

Information within the cell is not limited to genetic sequences or soluble signaling molecules. It is embedded in the composition and organization of lipids that define membranes. Each membrane encodes a set of physical conditions that determine how proteins behave, how signals propagate, and how the cell interprets its environment. This encoding is not symbolic. It is mechanical. Change the lipid composition and the behavior of receptors, channels, and enzymes shifts because the environment they operate in has been altered. Lipids therefore act as carriers of information by setting the constraints under which cellular processes occur.

The bilayer itself functions as a continuous input surface. Fatty acid chain length, degree of saturation, and headgroup composition determine packing density, curvature, and permeability. These properties influence how proteins insert into the membrane, how they move, and how they interact with one another. A membrane enriched in tightly packed lipids creates a different signaling landscape than one with greater disorder. Receptors embedded in these environments adopt different conformations and respond differently to the same ligand. The information is not in the ligand alone. It is in the structural context that defines how that ligand is processed.

Lipid diversity allows the cell to generate localized environments with distinct properties. Different regions of the same membrane can support different behaviors by varying lipid composition. This creates zones where specific processes are favored, such as signal initiation, transport, or mechanical stabilization. Proteins that require certain conditions localize to these regions, effectively reading the lipid environment as a set of instructions. When lipid composition changes, these instructions change, and proteins redistribute or alter their activity accordingly.

Signal transduction often begins with lipid modification. Enzymes alter specific lipids in response to external input, changing their structure and, in turn, the properties of the membrane. These changes can recruit proteins, alter membrane curvature, or modify permeability. The signal is carried through the membrane as a change in its physical state, not just as a cascade of soluble intermediates. This allows the cell to integrate information across a surface rather than relying solely on diffusion through the cytosol.

Time is encoded through lipid turnover. Membranes are continuously remodeled, with new lipids incorporated and existing ones modified or replaced. The rate and direction of this turnover determine how long a given state persists. Rapid turnover allows quick adaptation to changing conditions, while slower turnover stabilizes existing configurations. This creates a temporal dimension where the history of inputs influences current behavior through accumulated changes in membrane composition.

Lipid-mediated signaling extends beyond the cell surface. Internal membranes, including those of organelles, carry their own lipid compositions that define their function. Communication between compartments depends on how these membranes interact, fuse, or exchange material. The compatibility of lipid environments influences whether these interactions occur efficiently. Differences in composition act as barriers or gateways, controlling the flow of information within the cell.

Disturbance of lipid composition alters the information landscape. Changes in packing, curvature, or domain formation shift how signals are initiated and processed. The same external input can produce different outcomes because the membrane no longer presents the same structural conditions. This does not require changes in receptor number or ligand concentration. It arises from changes in the medium through which signaling occurs.

Lipids carry information by defining the architecture of the system. They determine how components are arranged, how they interact, and how signals are transmitted and resolved. The cell reads this information continuously, adjusting behavior based on the structural state of its membranes. Understanding signaling therefore requires understanding how lipid composition encodes and modifies the conditions under which all cellular processes operate.

Fatty Acids as Signaling Precursors

Fatty acids serve as stored signaling potential that can be released, transformed, and redeployed in response to changes at the membrane. They are not passive structural elements once incorporated into phospholipids. They are substrates held in reserve within the bilayer, positioned for rapid conversion into signaling molecules when enzymes act on specific sites. The membrane therefore functions as both a barrier and a reservoir, where the composition of fatty acids determines what signals can be generated and how quickly they can be produced.

Release begins with enzymatic cleavage. Phospholipases target defined positions on membrane phospholipids, liberating fatty acids that were previously constrained within the bilayer. The identity of the released fatty acid determines the signaling pathways that follow. Arachidonic acid, for example, enters a sequence of reactions that produce eicosanoids, which influence vascular tone, immune activity, and cellular stress responses. Other fatty acids follow different metabolic routes, producing signals with distinct effects. The membrane composition therefore sets the range of possible outputs before any stimulus occurs.

Conversion pathways define how these precursors are used. Once released, fatty acids are rapidly metabolized by enzymes that transform them into active signaling molecules. These transformations change the structure of the molecule, altering its interaction with receptors and its ability to diffuse through the cellular environment. The rate of conversion and the balance between competing pathways determine which signals dominate. If one pathway is favored, its products accumulate and shape the cellular response. If another pathway becomes more active, the profile of signals shifts accordingly.

Spatial control is maintained throughout this process. Enzymes responsible for release and conversion are localized to specific regions of the membrane, ensuring that signaling occurs in defined areas. This localization allows the cell to generate signals where they are needed rather than uniformly across the membrane. The proximity of enzymes to their substrates reduces delay and increases the precision of the response. Changes in membrane organization can disrupt this arrangement, altering where and how signals are produced.

The physical properties of fatty acids influence their signaling behavior. Chain length and degree of saturation affect how these molecules interact with enzymes and receptors. More unsaturated fatty acids are more flexible and can adopt conformations that facilitate interaction with a broader range of proteins. More saturated fatty acids are more rigid, influencing how they are processed and how they integrate into signaling pathways. These structural differences translate into functional differences in how signals are generated and how long they persist.

Signal termination depends on further metabolism and reintegration. Once fatty acid-derived signals have exerted their effects, they are broken down or re-esterified into membrane lipids. This restores the reservoir and resets the system for future signaling events. The efficiency of this process determines how quickly the system can return to baseline. If termination is delayed, signals persist and overlap with new inputs, increasing noise. If termination is efficient, signals remain discrete and controlled.

The balance of fatty acids within the membrane determines the baseline signaling capacity of the cell. A membrane enriched in specific fatty acids will produce a different set of signals than one with a different composition. This balance is not static. It changes over time as new fatty acids are incorporated and existing ones are modified. These changes alter the signaling potential of the system, influencing how the cell responds to future stimuli.

Fatty acids act as signaling precursors by linking membrane composition to dynamic cellular responses. The cell does not generate signals from nothing. It draws from a pre-existing pool embedded within its structure. The nature of that pool determines the range, intensity, and duration of signaling events, making membrane composition a direct determinant of how information is generated and processed.

Eicosanoids and Local Control Systems

Eicosanoids are generated at the site of membrane disturbance and act within a constrained radius, shaping conditions locally rather than broadcasting signals across the entire system. Their production begins when specific fatty acids are released from membrane phospholipids and immediately enter enzymatic pathways embedded in the same or adjacent membrane regions. This tight coupling between release and conversion limits diffusion and ensures that the signal reflects the conditions at that exact location. The result is a control system that operates through localized adjustments in vascular tone, permeability, immune activity, and cellular behavior, all determined by the lipid composition present at the time of activation.

The pathways that produce eicosanoids compete for the same substrates. Once a fatty acid such as arachidonic acid is liberated, it can be directed into cyclooxygenase, lipoxygenase, or related enzymatic routes. Each pathway generates a distinct set of molecules with different effects on surrounding cells. The balance between these pathways determines whether the local environment shifts toward constriction or dilation, activation or resolution, recruitment or containment. This balance is not decided after the fact. It is set by enzyme availability, membrane organization, and the relative concentrations of precursor fatty acids embedded in the bilayer.

Localization defines both the strength and duration of the signal. Eicosanoids act on nearby receptors and are rapidly degraded or converted into less active forms, preventing widespread propagation. This rapid turnover allows the system to adjust conditions in real time without creating persistent systemic effects. When production is controlled and termination is efficient, the local environment can shift quickly and then return to baseline. If production exceeds termination capacity, signals persist longer than intended, extending their influence beyond the original site and altering neighboring regions.

Membrane composition determines what signals can be produced and how they behave once formed. Different fatty acids yield different classes of eicosanoids, each with specific effects on cellular function. The proportion of these fatty acids within the membrane sets the baseline signaling profile. A shift in composition changes the distribution of signals generated during activation, altering how the local control system responds to the same stimulus. This does not require changes in receptor expression or enzyme levels. It arises from the available substrates embedded within the membrane.

Receptor interaction translates these signals into action. Eicosanoids bind to specific receptors on nearby cells, initiating changes in ion flux, enzyme activity, and gene expression. These effects alter vascular diameter, immune cell behavior, and tissue permeability. Because the signals are produced and act within a confined space, the response remains targeted. Cells outside this region remain unaffected unless the signal persists long enough or spreads far enough to reach them.

Structural integrity of the membrane influences the precision of this system. When lipid organization supports controlled release and conversion, signals are generated where needed and terminated when their function is complete. When membrane structure is unstable, release becomes less regulated, and conversion pathways may shift unpredictably. This produces overlapping signals with competing effects, increasing variability in the local response. The system remains active, but it loses clarity and control.

Eicosanoids function as a local control layer embedded within the membrane. They translate structural conditions into immediate adjustments in the surrounding environment, allowing the cell and its neighbors to respond to changes without relying on distant signaling systems. Their behavior reflects the composition and organization of the membrane because that structure determines both the inputs and the pathways available for signal generation.

Structural Origin of Inflammatory Signaling

Inflammatory signaling begins as a consequence of altered membrane structure rather than as an isolated biochemical decision. The membrane defines baseline conditions for containment, separation, and controlled exchange. When those conditions shift, either through mechanical disruption, oxidative modification, or changes in lipid composition, the system detects a loss of structural integrity and initiates a response. This response is not triggered by abstract signaling intent. It emerges from changes in packing density, permeability, and domain organization that alter how proteins behave and how molecules move across the boundary.

Disruption of lipid packing is the first event that changes signaling behavior. Tightly packed membranes restrict movement and maintain separation between compartments. When packing loosens, transient spaces within the bilayer increase, allowing ions and small molecules to pass in ways that were previously constrained. This alters local concentrations and electrical conditions, which directly affects membrane-bound proteins. Channels open under different thresholds, receptors adopt different conformations, and enzymes encounter substrates at rates that deviate from baseline. These changes create the initial conditions that favor activation of inflammatory pathways.

Fatty acid composition determines the type of signals that follow. Membranes enriched with certain fatty acids provide substrates that can be rapidly converted into signaling molecules when released.

Enzymatic cleavage of these lipids produces precursors that enter pathways generating eicosanoids and related compounds. The identity and proportion of these fatty acids set the profile of signals that will be produced. A shift in composition alters the balance between pathways, changing whether the local environment favors recruitment of immune cells, alteration of vascular tone, or resolution of the response.

Reactive byproducts reinforce structural disruption. When electron leakage or other processes generate reactive species, these molecules interact with membrane lipids, modifying their structure and further reducing packing stability. Oxidized lipids change how the bilayer behaves, increasing permeability and altering domain formation. This creates a feedback loop where initial disruption leads to chemical modification, which then amplifies the structural changes that initiated the response. The membrane becomes both the source and the target of the signaling process.

Protein localization changes as structure degrades. Receptors and enzymes that rely on ordered domains for proper positioning become dispersed or misaligned. This alters how they interact, increasing the likelihood of unintended activation. Proteins that are normally separated may come into contact, initiating pathways that would not be active under stable conditions. At the same time, proteins that require clustering for proper function may fail to assemble, weakening coordinated responses. The result is a mixture of activation and dysfunction driven by loss of spatial control.

Mechanical stress contributes to this process by altering membrane tension. Stretching or deformation changes how lipids pack and how proteins embedded within the membrane behave. Mechanosensitive channels respond to these changes by altering ion flow, which further modifies intracellular conditions. This links physical forces directly to biochemical signaling, integrating structural disruption with cellular response. The membrane translates mechanical input into chemical output through changes in its own organization.

Signal propagation depends on whether the structural changes are contained or spread. Localized disruption produces localized signaling, allowing targeted responses that can be resolved once the structure is restored. Widespread disruption extends these signals across larger regions, increasing the scale and duration of the response. The difference lies in how stable the surrounding membrane remains and whether it can prevent the spread of altered conditions.

Resolution requires restoration of structure. Lipid repair, replacement, and reorganization return the membrane to a state that supports controlled exchange and stable protein localization. As packing density increases and permeability decreases, the conditions that supported inflammatory signaling are removed. Signals diminish not because they are actively suppressed in isolation, but because the structural environment that allowed them to persist no longer exists.

Inflammatory signaling originates from changes in the material state of the membrane. It reflects how the system responds when the boundary that defines cellular organization is altered. The specific pathways that activate are determined by the available substrates and enzymes, but the initiation of the process is structural. Restore the structure and the signaling resolves as a consequence of returning the system to a stable operating condition.

Signal Timing and Termination

Signal timing is set by how quickly components assemble into a functional complex and how long that complex is held in place by the membrane. Initiation begins when receptors encounter ligands within a domain that supports clustering. The rate of that encounter is determined by lateral mobility and local density. When the membrane allows controlled movement, receptors find one another and assemble within a defined window, producing a signal with a sharp onset. If mobility is excessive, components fail to remain in contact long enough to stabilize the active state, delaying or weakening initiation. If mobility is too restricted, encounters occur slowly, stretching the onset over time and reducing responsiveness to changing input.

Propagation depends on maintaining proximity across sequential steps. Kinases, adaptors, and downstream effectors must bind in order, each interaction occurring before the previous one dissipates. The membrane enforces this sequence by confining these components within domains where interaction rates are high. When domains are intact, the signal moves forward with minimal delay because each step occurs within a localized environment. When domains fragment, components disperse between steps, increasing the time required for the next interaction and raising the chance that the signal will decay before completion. Timing becomes variable because the structure no longer holds the sequence together.

Amplitude and duration are linked through retention. A cluster that persists allows repeated interactions, reinforcing the signal and extending its duration. This persistence is not indefinite. It depends on the balance between forces that stabilize the cluster and processes that drive disassembly. Lipid composition sets this balance by determining how tightly components are packed and how easily they can separate. Stable packing supports sustained interaction long enough for full signal transmission. Instability shortens retention, truncating the signal before downstream pathways are fully engaged.

Termination requires coordinated disassembly and deactivation within the same spatial context where activation occurred. Phosphatases, lipid-modifying enzymes, and receptor internalization machinery must access the active complex while it is still localized. The membrane facilitates this by positioning termination components near activation sites. When this arrangement holds, signals end cleanly. Receptors return to baseline, and downstream molecules are reset. If activation and termination are separated spatially due to domain disruption, deactivation lags behind initiation. Signals persist beyond their intended duration, overlapping with new inputs and increasing noise.

Chemical gradients contribute to timing by controlling how quickly signaling intermediates are removed or converted. Molecules generated at the membrane must either diffuse away, be degraded, or be re-incorporated into the membrane. The rate of these processes determines how long the signal remains active. Efficient clearance shortens duration and sharpens resolution. Slower clearance extends duration and increases the likelihood of interaction with unrelated pathways. Membrane permeability and domain integrity influence these rates by controlling diffusion paths and access to enzymes.

Electrical conditions also shape timing. Changes in membrane potential alter the behavior of voltage-sensitive proteins, shifting activation thresholds and affecting how long channels remain open. Stable potential supports predictable timing, while fluctuations introduce variability in both onset and termination. Ion fluxes that respond to these changes feed back into the system, influencing enzyme activity and further modifying signal duration.

Signal timing and termination are therefore structural outcomes. The membrane defines how quickly components assemble, how long they remain together, and how efficiently they are dismantled. When structure supports controlled assembly and coordinated disassembly, signals begin and end with precision. When structure degrades, initiation becomes delayed or inconsistent, and termination becomes incomplete or prolonged. The system continues to process input, but without clear boundaries in time, leading to overlapping signals and reduced clarity in output.

Chapter 6

Inflammation as a Structural Event

Inflammation begins when the membrane no longer maintains the conditions required for controlled exchange and stable signaling. It is not initiated as a standalone program. It emerges when the boundary that defines the cell shifts in permeability, packing, and organization. These changes alter ion gradients, protein positioning, and the availability of signaling substrates, producing a coordinated response that reflects the state of the structure. The system reacts because the physical conditions that support normal operation have been disrupted, and restoration of those conditions becomes the priority.

Loss of packing density increases permeability and changes electrical balance. Ions that were previously contained move more freely, altering local charge and affecting voltage-sensitive channels. Calcium entry rises, triggering enzyme systems that respond to changes in intracellular concentration. These enzymes act on membrane lipids, releasing fatty acids that feed directly into signaling pathways. The sequence is continuous. Structural change alters ion movement, which activates enzymes, which then generate signals that further modify the local environment.

Domain organization breaks down as the membrane destabilizes. Regions that previously concentrated receptors and signaling proteins lose their integrity, dispersing components across the membrane. This changes interaction patterns. Some pathways fail to initiate because clustering cannot be sustained, while others activate inappropriately due to new proximities between proteins that are normally separated. The result is a shift from controlled signaling to a mixture of activation and interference, where outputs are less specific and more variable.

Fatty acid release provides the substrate for immediate local signaling. Phospholipases respond to changes in calcium and membrane state, liberating fatty acids that enter enzymatic pathways producing eicosanoids and related molecules. These signals act within the surrounding area, altering vascular tone, permeability, and immune cell behavior. The profile of these signals depends on the fatty acids present in the membrane at the time of activation. The membrane therefore determines not only that a response occurs, but also the type of response that is generated.

Reactive species reinforce the process by modifying membrane components. As electron leakage and enzymatic reactions increase, reactive molecules interact with lipids, changing their structure and further reducing packing stability. This increases permeability and accelerates domain disruption. The membrane becomes progressively less capable of maintaining gradients and organizing signaling components, amplifying the conditions that sustain the inflammatory response.

Mechanical stress integrates with these changes. Deformation of the membrane alters tension and curvature, influencing how lipids pack and how embedded proteins respond. Mechanosensitive channels open under these conditions, further altering ion flux and reinforcing the signaling cascade. Physical and chemical changes converge, each reinforcing the other as the system moves away from its stable state.

Signal propagation depends on the extent of structural disruption. Localized changes produce localized responses that can be resolved once membrane integrity is restored. Widespread disruption extends these signals across larger areas, increasing both intensity and duration. The scale of inflammation therefore reflects how broadly membrane structure has been altered and how effectively surrounding regions can maintain stability.

Resolution requires rebuilding the membrane. Lipids must be replaced, domains must reform, and permeability must return to controlled levels. As structure is restored, ion gradients stabilize, enzyme activity normalizes, and signaling pathways return to baseline. The inflammatory response subsides because the conditions that sustained it no longer exist. This is not a separate process. It is the continuation of structural repair reaching a point where the system can resume controlled operation.

Inflammation, viewed through this framework, is the system responding to structural failure at the membrane level. The pathways involved are known, but their activation is determined by the physical state of the membrane that houses them. When that state is stable, signaling remains controlled. When it is not, the same components generate a response aimed at restoring the boundary conditions required for normal function.

Membrane Damage as the Trigger

The initiating event is a change in the physical state of the membrane that alters containment, not a discrete biochemical switch. When packing loosens or continuity is interrupted, permeability increases and the distribution of ions shifts immediately. Calcium moves along its gradient into the cell, raising local concentrations near the inner leaflet. This rise is not interpreted abstractly. It directly changes enzyme behavior. Calcium-sensitive phospholipases activate at the membrane surface and begin cleaving phospholipids, releasing fatty acids that feed into rapid conversion pathways. The signal begins as a consequence of altered flux across a compromised boundary.

Damage also exposes lipids and protein domains that are normally sequestered within the bilayer. These exposed structures interact differently with surrounding proteins and extracellular components, creating new binding opportunities that were not present under intact conditions. Receptors that depend on defined orientation within a stable bilayer shift conformation when the surrounding lipids are disrupted. This alters their activity thresholds and increases the likelihood of spontaneous or low-threshold activation. The same receptor population produces a different output because the structural constraints that held it in a specific state have changed.

Mechanical discontinuities propagate through the membrane plane. A localized defect alters tension in adjacent regions, changing how lipids pack and how proteins move. Mechanosensitive channels respond to these shifts by opening, further increasing ion flux and reinforcing the initial disturbance. This spreads the effect beyond the point of damage, creating a gradient of altered conditions that extends into neighboring domains. The signal therefore expands from a structural defect into a broader field of modified membrane behavior.

Reactive modification follows quickly. Increased ion flux and disrupted electron flow generate reactive species that interact with nearby lipids. Oxidized lipids change shape and packing characteristics, introducing further instability into the bilayer. These changes increase permeability and disrupt domain organization, making it more difficult for the membrane to re-establish its original state. The system enters a reinforcing cycle where structural damage promotes chemical modification, and chemical modification deepens structural disruption.

Transport processes shift as a result. Channels and carriers embedded in the membrane rely on stable gradients and consistent lipid environments. When these conditions change, transport rates alter in ways that can either amplify or partially compensate for the disturbance. In many cases, the increased permeability overrides controlled transport, allowing passive movement to dominate. This reduces the system's ability to maintain separation between compartments, further eroding the conditions required for controlled signaling.

The immediate consequence is the generation of local signals derived from the membrane itself. Released fatty acids are converted into short-lived mediators that act on nearby cells and structures. These mediators adjust vascular tone, permeability, and immune cell positioning, all within the region defined by the original structural change. The response is proportional to the extent of the damage because the amount of released substrate and the degree of altered flux scale with the size of the disruption.

Containment determines whether the response remains localized or spreads. If surrounding membrane regions retain their integrity, they limit the propagation of altered conditions and confine signaling to the site of damage. If adjacent regions are already unstable, the disturbance extends outward, producing a larger field of activation. The membrane either isolates the event or allows it to expand depending on its baseline condition.

Membrane damage functions as the trigger because it directly alters the parameters that govern ion movement, enzyme activation, and protein behavior. The subsequent signaling pathways are engaged because the structural environment has shifted, not because a separate decision has been made. Restoration of the membrane reverses these conditions. Ion gradients re-establish, enzyme activity returns to baseline, and the signals generated from the disruption diminish as the boundary regains its capacity to contain and organize the system.

Omega-6 and Omega-3 Balance as Substrate Competition

The balance between omega-6 and omega-3 fatty acids is determined at the level of the membrane as a question of occupancy and access. Both classes are incorporated into phospholipids and held within the bilayer as potential substrates. When activation occurs and phospholipases release fatty acids, these substrates compete for the same enzymatic pathways. The outcome is not decided after release. It is largely predetermined by which fatty acids are present in the membrane and in what proportion. The system draws from what is already embedded in its structure, so composition sets the direction of signaling before any stimulus is applied.

Once released, these fatty acids enter shared conversion routes. Cyclooxygenase and lipoxygenase enzymes do not selectively process one class in isolation. They act on available substrates, and the relative abundance of each determines which products are generated in greater quantity. Omega-6-derived substrates tend to produce signaling molecules that promote vascular constriction, increased permeability, and immune cell recruitment. Omega-3-derived substrates enter pathways that yield signals associated with controlled resolution, reduction of excessive permeability, and restoration of baseline conditions. These outputs are not opposites in an abstract sense. They represent different structural responses to changes in the membrane environment.

Competition occurs at multiple stages. It begins with incorporation into the membrane, where both omega-6 and omega-3 fatty acids occupy positions within phospholipids. It continues during release, where enzymes act on available lipids without preference beyond accessibility. It persists through conversion, where enzymes process whichever substrate is most available at that moment. At each stage, the relative presence of these fatty acids determines which pathways dominate. A membrane enriched in one class will produce a corresponding profile of signaling molecules because those substrates are more likely to be released and converted.

The physical properties of these fatty acids also influence how they behave within the membrane. Differences in chain structure affect packing, fluidity, and the formation of domains. These structural effects alter enzyme access and protein localization, indirectly shaping which substrates are processed. A membrane with altered packing characteristics may expose certain fatty acids more readily or position enzymes in a way that favors one pathway over another. The competition is therefore both chemical and structural, governed by how these molecules are arranged within the bilayer.

Signal duration and termination are affected by the same balance. Products derived from different substrates have different lifespans and rates of degradation. If one class dominates, its signaling molecules persist and shape the local environment for longer periods. This influences how quickly the system can return to baseline after activation. Efficient resolution depends on the availability of substrates that support pathways leading to termination and repair. If those substrates are limited, signals associated with activation continue to dominate, extending the response.

The balance between omega-6 and omega-3 fatty acids does not act as a simple ratio in isolation. It reflects the composition of the membrane and the distribution of substrates within it. Changes in this balance alter the set of signals that can be generated, the rate at which they are produced, and how long they persist. The system does not choose between pathways independently of structure. It follows the constraints imposed by the substrates available within the membrane at the time of activation.

Substrate competition therefore defines the direction of local signaling by determining which pathways receive input under conditions of activation. The membrane acts as the source of these inputs, and its composition dictates the outcome before enzymatic processing begins. Adjusting this composition changes the signaling landscape by altering which substrates are available to compete, thereby shifting the profile of responses generated when the system is engaged.

Resolution Pathways and Failure to Complete

Resolution is not a passive fade-out of signaling. It is an organized sequence that depends on a shift in membrane-derived substrates, reassembly of domains, and restoration of controlled flux across the boundary. Once the initiating disturbance has been contained, the system must transition from generating activation signals to producing mediators that terminate the response and rebuild structure. This transition is constrained by what remains in the membrane. If the lipid environment supports the generation of resolving mediators, the system proceeds toward completion. If it does not, the initial response continues to cycle because the conditions required to terminate it are absent.

The switch begins at the level of substrate use. As activation progresses, the pool of released fatty acids is redirected into pathways that generate resolving molecules rather than additional pro-activation signals. This redirection requires both the presence of appropriate substrates and the positioning of enzymes that convert them. When these elements are aligned, local signaling shifts from increasing permeability and recruitment to tightening the boundary and clearing accumulated intermediates. Vascular tone normalizes, immune activity contracts to the site of need, and excess signaling molecules are degraded or re-incorporated into the membrane.

Spatial organization determines whether this transition occurs cleanly. Enzymes responsible for resolution must operate in the same regions where activation took place. If domain structure is intact, these enzymes access substrates efficiently and terminate signals at their point of origin. When domains are unstable, substrates and enzymes are no longer co-localized. Activation pathways continue because their components remain active, while resolution pathways lag due to loss of access. This creates a mismatch where initiation outpaces termination, extending the duration of the response.

Termination also requires restoration of ion gradients and electrical stability. As membrane permeability decreases and packing improves, ion flux returns to controlled pathways. Calcium levels fall, reducing activation of phospholipases and other enzymes that drive signal generation. This shift reduces the release of new substrates and allows existing signals to decay. If permeability remains elevated, ion flux continues to stimulate activation pathways, preventing the system from exiting the response state. The membrane remains in a condition that supports continued signaling rather than completion.

Failure to complete arises when structural repair does not keep pace with signaling demand. Damaged lipids persist, domain organization remains fragmented, and gradients cannot be fully re-established. Under these conditions, resolving pathways are present but insufficient. Signals that should terminate are replaced by new signals generated from ongoing structural instability. The system appears to be active continuously because the trigger condition has not been removed. Each attempt at resolution is interrupted by new inputs generated from the same compromised membrane.

Reactive byproducts reinforce this failure. Oxidative modification of lipids alters their behavior and reduces the ability of the membrane to return to a tightly packed state. These modified lipids can continue to serve as substrates for signaling, extending the response. At the same time, they impair the formation of domains required for coordinated termination. The system becomes trapped in a cycle where structural damage sustains signaling, and signaling contributes to further structural disruption.

Clearance mechanisms depend on the same structural conditions. Cells and enzymes responsible for removing debris and resolving intermediates must operate within a stable environment to function efficiently. When the membrane remains unstable, these processes slow or become misdirected. Accumulated intermediates persist, interacting with surrounding components and maintaining activation. The boundary is not restored, so the system does not return to baseline.

Completion requires that the membrane re-establish its role as a controlled barrier. Lipid composition must shift toward configurations that support tight packing, domain formation, and stable gradients. As this occurs, substrate release declines, resolving mediators dominate, and signaling pathways shut down in sequence. The response ends because the structural conditions that sustained it have been removed.

Resolution pathways succeed when structure is restored faster than new disruption occurs. They fail when the membrane remains in a state that continuously generates signals. The difference is not in the presence of resolving mechanisms, but in whether the underlying architecture allows those mechanisms to operate to completion.

Chronic Inflammation as Incomplete Signaling

Chronic inflammation reflects a system that initiates a response but cannot carry it through to termination because the structural conditions required for completion are never restored. The membrane remains in a state that continues to generate activation signals while simultaneously impairing the pathways that would normally shut those signals down. The result is not a constant high-level response, but a persistent cycle of partial activation, failed resolution, and reactivation driven by the same underlying instability.

The process begins with a disturbance that alters membrane packing, permeability, and domain organization. Ion gradients shift, calcium levels rise, and enzymes release fatty acids that enter signaling pathways. Under normal conditions, this sequence would transition into resolution as membrane integrity is repaired. In the chronic state, repair does not reach a level that restores containment. Permeability remains elevated, allowing continued ion flux that sustains enzyme activation. Each attempt to terminate the signal is interrupted by new inputs generated from the same compromised structure.

Substrate availability reinforces this cycle. The membrane continues to supply fatty acids that feed into activation pathways, while the substrates required for resolution are either insufficient or not effectively converted due to disrupted enzyme localization. The balance remains tilted toward ongoing signal generation. Even when resolving mediators are produced, they are outpaced by new signals because the source of activation has not been removed. The system attempts to complete the response, but the conditions necessary for completion are not present.

Domain instability contributes to the persistence of signaling. Without stable regions to localize receptors, enzymes, and termination machinery, interactions occur without coordination. Activation pathways may initiate in one region while termination processes are delayed or displaced. Signals overlap and extend beyond their intended duration because the spatial organization required for clean sequencing is absent. The system operates with reduced precision, where timing becomes inconsistent and signals fail to resolve into discrete events.

Electrical instability adds another layer. Fluctuations in membrane potential alter the behavior of channels and receptors, shifting activation thresholds and prolonging signaling states. Ion transport systems respond to these fluctuations, but their adjustments cannot stabilize the environment if the underlying membrane remains permeable. The system compensates continuously, but compensation does not equal restoration. Energy is expended to maintain function, yet the baseline condition remains altered.

Reactive modification maintains the structural defect. Lipids exposed to ongoing stress are oxidized or otherwise altered, preventing the reformation of tightly packed domains. These modified lipids continue to influence membrane behavior, sustaining permeability and disrupting protein localization. The membrane becomes a persistent source of activation because its composition no longer supports the conditions required for termination.

Chronic inflammation therefore represents incomplete signaling. The initiation phase proceeds, but the resolution phase cannot fully engage because the structural framework that supports it is compromised. Signals are generated, partially processed, and then renewed before they can be cleared. The system remains active not because it is intentionally sustaining the response, but because it cannot reach the structural state that would allow the response to end.

Restoring completion requires restoring the membrane as a controlled boundary. Packing density must increase, domains must reform, and ion gradients must stabilize. As these conditions return, activation pathways lose their continuous input, and termination mechanisms regain access to their targets. The signaling cycle can then proceed from initiation to completion without interruption, allowing the system to return to baseline rather than remaining in a state of persistent partial activation.

Chapter 7

Hormonal Signaling and Membrane State

Hormonal signaling is constrained by the membrane that receives, organizes, and transmits the signal. Hormones arrive as inputs, but the output they generate depends on how receptors are positioned, how they move, and how they interact with downstream machinery within the lipid environment. The membrane defines these conditions by controlling packing density, domain formation, and electrical stability. When structure supports alignment, hormonal signals produce coordinated responses. When structure is altered, the same hormone produces a different output because the context that governs receptor behavior has shifted.

Receptors are not isolated sensors. They are embedded components whose activity depends on their surrounding lipids. Membrane composition determines receptor conformation, influencing how easily it transitions between inactive and active states. In tightly organized regions, receptors cluster and interact with co-receptors and signaling proteins in a controlled manner. Ligand binding leads to coordinated activation across multiple receptors, producing a signal that can propagate efficiently. When the membrane lacks this organization, receptors remain dispersed, and activation events fail to combine into a unified output. The hormone is present, but the signal does not scale because the structure does not support amplification.

Mobility within the membrane sets responsiveness. Receptors must move laterally to encounter partners and form signaling complexes. Adequate mobility allows rapid assembly when a hormone binds, producing a timely response. Excessive mobility prevents stable interactions, causing complexes to dissolve before the signal can propagate. Restricted mobility delays assembly, reducing sensitivity to changes in hormone concentration. The membrane defines this balance, determining how quickly and how reliably hormonal signals are processed.

Domain organization directs specificity. Different hormones rely on distinct receptor systems that must remain separated to avoid interference. Lipid domains create these separations by concentrating compatible components and excluding others. This ensures that each signaling pathway operates within its own defined region. When domains are stable, signals remain specific, and cross-talk is minimized. When domains fragment, components from different pathways mix, leading to overlapping or conflicting signals. The system becomes less precise because the structural boundaries that enforce separation have degraded.

Electrical properties influence receptor activation and downstream signaling. Many hormone receptors and associated channels respond to changes in membrane potential. A stable electrical environment supports predictable activation thresholds and consistent signaling dynamics. When permeability increases and potential fluctuates, these thresholds shift. Receptors may activate at lower or higher input levels, and signaling duration may extend or shorten unpredictably. Ion fluxes that accompany these changes further influence intracellular pathways, integrating electrical instability with biochemical signaling.

Hormone sensitivity is therefore not fixed. It emerges from the interaction between hormone concentration and membrane state. A well-structured membrane can produce strong responses to modest inputs because receptors are positioned and organized to amplify the signal. A disorganized membrane requires higher input to achieve the same effect and may still produce inconsistent output. This alters how the system interprets hormonal signals, affecting processes that depend on precise regulation.

Termination of hormonal signaling depends on the same structural conditions. Receptors must disengage, complexes must disassemble, and downstream pathways must reset. This requires coordinated access of termination mechanisms within the membrane. When structure supports this coordination, signals end cleanly. When it does not, activation persists or overlaps with new inputs, increasing variability in response.

Hormonal signaling is therefore an expression of membrane state. The hormone provides the input, but the membrane determines how that input is translated into output. Changes in lipid composition, domain stability, and permeability alter the behavior of receptors and the pathways they control. The system responds not only to the presence of hormones, but to the structural conditions that define how those hormones are processed.

Receptor Sensitivity as a Membrane-Dependent Property

Receptor sensitivity is set by the physical environment in which the receptor is embedded, not by receptor number alone. The membrane determines how easily a receptor transitions into its active state, how long that state is maintained, and how effectively it engages downstream partners. Lipid packing, domain organization, and local electrical conditions define the baseline from which a receptor responds to input. Change those conditions and the same receptor population produces a different response to the same hormone concentration.

Conformation depends on surrounding lipids. Receptors span the bilayer and interact directly with lipid headgroups and acyl chains. These interactions influence the shape of the receptor and the stability of its active and inactive states. In a tightly packed environment, the receptor is constrained, and activation requires sufficient input to overcome that constraint. Once activated, the same environment can stabilize the active conformation if clustering occurs within a compatible domain. In a more disordered membrane, the receptor experiences less constraint, lowering the threshold for activation but also reducing stability. Activation becomes easier but less controlled, and signals are more likely to fluctuate.

Clustering amplifies sensitivity by increasing local receptor density. When receptors are organized within domains, ligand binding to one receptor increases the likelihood that neighboring receptors will also engage. This produces a coordinated response that scales with input. The membrane enables this by supporting lateral movement within defined regions and by concentrating compatible proteins. When domains are disrupted, receptors remain dispersed, and activation events do not combine. Sensitivity decreases because higher input is required to achieve the same level of coordinated activation.

Coupling to downstream pathways depends on proximity and alignment. Receptors must interact with specific proteins to transmit a signal. The membrane positions these components so that interaction occurs rapidly after activation. If the membrane maintains this organization, signaling proceeds efficiently. If components are misaligned due to changes in lipid composition or domain structure, the receptor may activate without successfully engaging downstream machinery. This creates a state where binding occurs, but signal transmission is weak or incomplete.

Electrical conditions modify sensitivity further. Changes in membrane potential influence the behavior of voltage-sensitive receptors and associated channels. Stable potential supports consistent activation thresholds, allowing predictable responses to input. Fluctuating potential shifts these thresholds, altering how receptors respond to the same signal. Ion fluxes that accompany these changes feed back into receptor behavior, reinforcing or dampening sensitivity depending on the direction of change.

Desensitization and resensitization are also membrane-dependent processes. After activation, receptors must be reset to respond again. This involves disassembly of signaling complexes, internalization, or conformational changes that return the receptor to its baseline state. The membrane controls how quickly and efficiently this occurs by governing access of regulatory proteins and the mobility required for receptor trafficking. When structure supports coordinated disassembly, receptors reset cleanly. When structure is compromised, receptors may remain partially active or fail to return to a responsive state, reducing overall sensitivity.

Receptor sensitivity emerges from the interaction between receptor structure and membrane environment. It reflects how the membrane constrains movement, organizes interactions, and maintains electrical and chemical stability. Adjustments to membrane composition change these conditions, altering how receptors interpret and respond to signals. The system does not rely solely on receptor abundance to regulate sensitivity. It relies on the structural context that determines how those receptors behave under varying inputs.

Insulin Signaling and Membrane Composition

Insulin signaling begins at the membrane but is determined by whether that membrane can organize and stabilize the insulin receptor and its downstream machinery under load. The insulin receptor is a transmembrane tyrosine kinase that requires precise positioning and clustering to transition from ligand binding to effective signal propagation. The lipid environment defines how easily this transition occurs. Packing density, domain formation, and local electrical conditions set the threshold for activation and the efficiency of downstream coupling. When the membrane supports alignment, insulin binding produces a coordinated cascade that moves glucose transporters to the surface and shifts cellular metabolism. When it does not, binding occurs but signal transmission is incomplete or delayed.

Receptor activation depends on proximity and orientation. Insulin binding promotes autophosphorylation of the receptor, which requires that receptor subunits are correctly aligned within the membrane. Lipid composition influences this alignment by controlling how the receptor sits within the bilayer and how it interacts with neighboring receptors. In membranes that support domain formation, receptors are concentrated into regions where interaction probability is high. This increases the likelihood that activation will propagate beyond the initial binding event. In membranes that lack this organization, receptors remain dispersed, and activation remains localized, reducing the strength of the signal.

Downstream signaling requires rapid recruitment of adaptor proteins and kinases to the receptor. These components must encounter the activated receptor within a defined time window to propagate the signal. The membrane governs this process by controlling lateral mobility and spatial confinement. When mobility is balanced with stability, adaptor proteins are recruited efficiently, and the signal proceeds through the pathway without delay. If mobility is excessive, components fail to remain in contact long enough to transmit the signal. If mobility is restricted, recruitment is slowed, and the signal weakens before it can be amplified.

Membrane composition also influences the formation of lipid domains that support insulin signaling. Certain lipids promote environments where signaling complexes can assemble and remain stable long enough to complete their function. These domains act as platforms where the receptor, its substrates, and downstream enzymes are co-localized. When these platforms are intact, signaling proceeds with precision. When they are disrupted, components disperse, and the pathway becomes less efficient, requiring higher insulin levels to achieve the same effect.

Glucose transporter translocation depends on this structural framework. After activation, signaling pathways direct vesicles containing glucose transporters to the membrane. Fusion of these vesicles requires membrane regions that can accommodate curvature and maintain integrity during the process. Lipid composition determines whether these regions form and whether fusion occurs efficiently. If the membrane lacks the necessary properties, transporter insertion is reduced, limiting glucose uptake even when upstream signaling is partially active.

Electrical and ionic conditions further modify insulin signaling. Changes in membrane potential and ion gradients influence the activity of kinases and other signaling proteins involved in the pathway. Stable conditions support consistent signaling, while fluctuations introduce variability in activation and propagation. Increased permeability or disrupted gradients alter how these proteins behave, contributing to reduced signaling efficiency.

Insulin resistance emerges when membrane conditions no longer support coordinated signaling. The receptor may still bind insulin, but clustering is reduced, adaptor recruitment is impaired, and transporter translocation is inefficient. The system compensates by increasing insulin levels, but this does not restore the structural conditions required for efficient signaling. The outcome is reduced responsiveness despite the presence of adequate or elevated input.

Membrane composition therefore determines how insulin signaling is executed. It sets the conditions for receptor activation, pathway propagation, and final functional output. Changes in lipid organization alter each stage of the process, shifting the system from coordinated response to partial or inconsistent signaling because the structural framework required for efficient communication is no longer maintained.

Steroid Hormone Interaction with Lipid Environments

Steroid hormones do not approach the cell as purely external signals. Their structure allows them to partition directly into the lipid phase, making the membrane both an entry point and an active participant in how the signal is processed. Before a receptor is engaged, the hormone has already interacted with the bilayer, and that interaction is shaped by lipid composition, packing density, and domain organization. The membrane determines how readily the molecule inserts, how it distributes within the bilayer, and how efficiently it reaches its intracellular targets.

Partitioning depends on compatibility with the lipid environment. Steroid molecules align with the hydrophobic core of the membrane, positioning themselves among fatty acid chains. In membranes with tighter packing, insertion is more constrained, and movement through the bilayer is slower but more controlled. In more disordered membranes, insertion occurs with less resistance, but distribution becomes less predictable, and the hormone may diffuse unevenly across regions. This affects how uniformly receptors are engaged and how consistent the resulting signal will be across the cell.

Movement through the membrane is not uniform. Lipid domains create regions where diffusion rates differ, altering the path a steroid hormone takes as it traverses the bilayer. Ordered domains can slow movement and concentrate the molecule in specific regions, increasing the likelihood of interaction with localized receptors or transport mechanisms. Less ordered regions allow faster diffusion but reduce the probability of sustained interaction with any single receptor system. The membrane therefore guides the hormone toward certain signaling routes while limiting others, based on its internal organization.

Receptor engagement depends on how the hormone exits the membrane and encounters its binding site. Many steroid hormone receptors are located within the cytosol or nucleus, requiring the hormone to cross the bilayer and enter the intracellular environment. The efficiency of this transition is influenced by membrane permeability and the stability of the lipid barrier. If the membrane is too rigid, passage slows, delaying signal initiation. If it is too permeable, the hormone may diffuse rapidly but without controlled distribution, leading to uneven receptor activation.

Membrane composition also affects the availability and behavior of membrane-associated steroid receptors. Some receptors are embedded within or closely associated with the membrane, responding to hormones that remain within the lipid phase. These receptors depend on local lipid conditions to maintain their conformation and interaction with signaling partners. Changes in lipid composition alter how these receptors function, shifting their sensitivity and the pathways they activate.

Steroid hormones can modify the membrane as they pass through it. Their presence within the bilayer alters local packing and can influence the behavior of nearby lipids and proteins. This creates a feedback effect where the hormone not only responds to the membrane environment but also contributes to changes in that environment. These changes may be transient, but they can influence how subsequent signaling events unfold.

Electrical and chemical conditions intersect with these interactions. Changes in membrane potential and ion gradients can influence how steroid hormones partition and move, as well as how receptors respond once engaged. Stable conditions support predictable signaling, while fluctuations introduce variability in both hormone distribution and receptor activation.

The interaction between steroid hormones and lipid environments therefore precedes and shapes the signaling process. The membrane determines how the hormone enters, where it travels, and how effectively it engages its targets. Changes in lipid composition alter each of these steps, producing different outcomes from the same hormonal input because the structural medium through which the signal passes has been modified.

Hormonal Instability as Structural Drift

Hormonal instability reflects a gradual loss of membrane conditions that support consistent receptor behavior, signal propagation, and termination. The system does not fail because hormones disappear or receptors vanish. It becomes unstable because the lipid environment that governs how signals are processed drifts away from the state required for coordinated function. This drift alters thresholds, timing, and amplification, producing variable outputs from the same hormonal input.

The process begins with changes in lipid composition that affect packing and domain formation. As membranes shift toward less stable configurations, receptor positioning becomes less consistent. Clusters that once formed reliably now assemble intermittently or not at all. This changes the relationship between hormone concentration and response. At times, small inputs produce exaggerated effects when clusters form unexpectedly. At other times, larger inputs fail to generate sufficient activation because receptors remain dispersed. The signal becomes inconsistent because the structural conditions that define sensitivity are no longer stable.

Mobility within the membrane contributes to this variability. Receptors must move to interact with co-receptors and downstream proteins. When lipid organization drifts, this movement becomes either excessive or restricted depending on local conditions. Excessive movement prevents stable complex formation, shortening signal duration and reducing amplification. Restricted movement delays interaction, increasing the time required for activation and reducing responsiveness. The system shifts between these states as membrane properties fluctuate, producing irregular signaling patterns.

Domain instability disrupts pathway separation. Hormonal systems rely on distinct regions of the membrane to maintain specificity and prevent interference between pathways. As domains lose definition, components from different signaling systems begin to overlap. This creates cross-talk where signals intended for one pathway influence another. The result is a loss of clarity, where outputs reflect mixed inputs rather than discrete signaling events. Hormonal regulation becomes less precise because structural boundaries that enforce separation are weakened.

Electrical instability reinforces these effects. Changes in membrane permeability alter ion gradients and membrane potential, shifting activation thresholds for receptors and associated channels. Fluctuating potential changes how receptors respond to the same hormone level, producing variability in both onset and duration of signaling. Ion fluxes that accompany these changes influence intracellular pathways, adding another layer of inconsistency to the system.

Termination processes are affected in parallel. Receptors must disengage, complexes must disassemble, and signaling molecules must be cleared to reset the system. Structural drift interferes with these processes by dispersing termination machinery or altering the conditions required for deactivation. Signals persist longer than intended or fail to terminate cleanly, overlapping with new inputs. This accumulation of partially resolved signals contributes to instability, as the system never fully returns to baseline.

Transport and distribution of hormones are also influenced by membrane state. For hormones that interact with or pass through the membrane, changes in lipid composition alter how they partition and move. This affects how uniformly receptors are engaged across the cell. Uneven distribution leads to localized differences in signaling, further increasing variability in response.

Hormonal instability therefore emerges from a membrane that no longer enforces consistent conditions for signaling. The same inputs are present, but the system processes them differently over time because the structural framework that governs receptor behavior, interaction, and termination is in flux. Restoring stability requires restoring membrane composition and organization so that receptor systems operate within defined boundaries, allowing signals to be generated, propagated, and resolved with consistency rather than variability.

PART III

SYSTEM-LEVEL CONSEQUENCES OF LIPID DISTORTION

Chapter 8

Metabolic Instability

Metabolic instability emerges when the membrane can no longer coordinate the flow of substrates, electrons, and signals within defined boundaries. Metabolism depends on controlled movement across membranes, stable gradients, and organized enzyme systems that operate in sequence. When membrane structure drifts, these conditions fragment. Substrates arrive at the wrong rates, gradients fluctuate, and enzymatic pathways lose alignment. The system continues to process fuel, but it does so without coherence, producing variable output and increasing the cost of maintaining baseline function.

Fuel selection is altered at the level of transport. Entry of fatty acids, glucose, and other substrates depends on membrane carriers that operate under specific gradient and structural conditions. When permeability increases or gradients weaken, transport becomes less predictable. Some substrates enter too quickly, others too slowly, and the balance between fuel sources shifts. This imbalance changes how downstream pathways are engaged, forcing the system to compensate by redirecting metabolic flow in ways that are less efficient.

Mitochondrial function reflects these changes immediately. The inner membrane must maintain a proton gradient to couple electron transport to ATP production. Structural drift increases proton leakage, reducing the gradient and forcing the mitochondrion to increase substrate oxidation to maintain ATP output. This raises oxygen consumption and increases electron escape, generating reactive species that further damage membrane components. Energy production continues, but with reduced efficiency and increased byproduct formation, placing additional stress on the system.

Enzymatic pathways lose coordination when spatial organization breaks down. Many metabolic reactions depend on proximity between enzymes that pass intermediates from one step to the next. Membrane-associated domains help maintain this proximity. When domains fragment, intermediates diffuse away from their intended pathways, slowing reaction rates and increasing the likelihood of side reactions. The sequence of metabolism becomes less direct, requiring more input to achieve the same output.

Hormonal signaling that regulates metabolism is affected in parallel. Insulin, glucagon, and other hormones rely on membrane structure to produce consistent responses. When receptor sensitivity and signaling efficiency fluctuate, metabolic pathways are activated or suppressed inconsistently. Glucose uptake may not align with insulin levels, and lipid metabolism may not adjust appropriately to energy demand. The system loses its ability to match input with output because the signaling framework that coordinates these processes is unstable.

Ion gradients contribute to metabolic control by influencing enzyme activity and transport processes. Changes in membrane permeability alter these gradients, affecting how enzymes function and how substrates move between compartments. Calcium flux, in particular, links membrane state to mitochondrial activity, altering the rate of energy production in response to changes in cellular conditions. When gradients are unstable, these regulatory mechanisms become inconsistent, further disrupting metabolic coordination.

Accumulation of intermediates reflects this loss of control. When pathways are not aligned, substrates and partially processed molecules build up. These intermediates can interact with other pathways, producing additional byproducts and increasing metabolic noise. The system attempts to clear these accumulations, but without structural organization, clearance is less efficient, and accumulation persists.

Metabolic instability is therefore a structural problem expressed through biochemical output. The pathways remain intact, but the conditions required for their coordinated operation are compromised. Substrates, enzymes, and signals are present, yet their interactions are no longer synchronized. Restoring stability requires re-establishing membrane conditions that support controlled transport, stable gradients, and organized enzyme activity, allowing metabolism to proceed with coherence rather than fragmentation.

Fuel Handling as a Membrane-Dependent Process

Fuel handling is determined at the boundary where substrates encounter the membrane, not at the level of downstream pathways alone. Every molecule that enters, exits, or is redirected within the cell must cross or interact with a membrane whose structure sets the rules for movement. Transporters, channels, and passive diffusion all operate within constraints defined by lipid composition, packing, and electrical gradients. When these conditions are stable, fuel entry and distribution align with demand. When they are not, substrates move at rates and in patterns that disrupt coordination between intake, processing, and output.

Transporter behavior depends on the local membrane environment. Proteins responsible for moving glucose, fatty acids, and other substrates require specific lipid conditions to maintain their conformation and activity. The surrounding bilayer influences how these proteins open, close, and cycle between states. In a membrane that supports proper packing and domain organization, transporters function with predictable kinetics, allowing substrate flow to match metabolic needs. When the membrane becomes disordered, transporter activity becomes inconsistent. Some remain open longer than intended, increasing influx, while others fail to cycle efficiently, limiting availability of key substrates.

Gradient dependence links fuel handling to membrane integrity. Many transport processes rely on electrochemical gradients to drive movement. These gradients exist only if the membrane can maintain separation between compartments. Increased permeability reduces gradient strength, altering how substrates are transported. In some cases, transport slows because the driving force is diminished. In others, passive movement increases, bypassing regulated pathways and reducing control over substrate entry. The balance between controlled and uncontrolled movement shifts as membrane conditions change.

Partitioning within the membrane affects lipid-based fuels directly. Fatty acids and related molecules interact with the bilayer before entering metabolic pathways. Their distribution within the membrane determines how accessible they are to enzymes and transport systems. Lipid composition influences this distribution by altering packing and domain formation. A membrane that supports organized domains can concentrate specific lipid species in regions where they are efficiently processed. Disordered membranes disperse these molecules, reducing the efficiency of their utilization.

Coordination between different fuel sources depends on consistent signaling at the membrane. Hormonal inputs regulate which substrates are prioritized, but the membrane determines how these signals are executed. If receptor sensitivity and signaling pathways are stable, the system shifts between fuel sources in a controlled manner. If membrane structure is unstable, these signals are processed inconsistently, leading to mismatches between substrate availability and metabolic demand. The cell may take in fuel that it cannot process efficiently or fail to utilize available substrates when needed.

Storage and release of fuels are also influenced by membrane conditions. Lipid droplets and glycogen-associated processes interact with membranes that control access to stored substrates. Changes in membrane composition alter how these storage systems are mobilized, affecting the rate at which fuels are released into active pathways. This adds another layer where structural conditions determine whether the system can respond appropriately to changing energy requirements.

Fuel handling therefore reflects the state of the membrane at every stage. Entry, distribution, utilization, and storage are all governed by how well the membrane maintains gradients, organizes transporters, and supports signaling. When structure is intact, these processes align, allowing substrates to be handled in a coordinated and efficient manner. When structure drifts, the same components operate under altered conditions, producing variability in how fuels are managed because the boundary that defines their movement no longer enforces consistent control.

Glucose Dysregulation as Signaling Failure

Glucose dysregulation develops when the membrane can no longer translate hormonal input into coordinated transport and intracellular handling. The issue is not simply the presence of glucose or the amount of insulin in circulation. It is the failure of receptor activation, signal propagation, and transporter deployment to occur within a stable structural framework. The same inputs arrive, but the membrane no longer organizes the sequence required to move glucose from the extracellular space into controlled intracellular use.

The process begins at the insulin receptor. Binding alone does not ensure function. The receptor must align, cluster, and autophosphorylate in a membrane environment that supports these interactions. When lipid composition supports domain formation and controlled mobility, activation propagates efficiently to downstream proteins. When the membrane is disordered, receptors remain dispersed or form unstable clusters. Autophosphorylation occurs inconsistently, and the signal weakens before it can recruit adaptor proteins. The pathway initiates but does not reach the threshold required for full activation.

Propagation failure follows immediately. Insulin signaling depends on rapid recruitment of intermediates that transmit the signal toward glucose transporter mobilization. These intermediates must encounter the activated receptor within a defined window. Membrane instability alters encounter rates by changing mobility and spatial organization. Components either fail to meet in time or do not remain in contact long enough to sustain the signal. The result is partial activation that cannot drive the downstream processes required for effective glucose handling.

Transporter deployment reflects this breakdown. Vesicles containing glucose transporters must be directed to and fused with the membrane. Fusion requires specific membrane curvature, lipid composition, and local organization. When these conditions are intact, transporters insert into the membrane, increasing glucose uptake rapidly in response to insulin. When structure is compromised, vesicle docking and fusion are inefficient. Even if signaling upstream is partially active, transporter insertion is reduced, limiting glucose entry into the cell.

Electrical and ionic instability further disrupts this system. Changes in membrane potential and ion gradients alter kinase activity and signaling dynamics, shifting thresholds and timing. Calcium flux, which influences multiple steps in the signaling pathway, becomes less controlled. These changes introduce variability into both activation and transporter deployment, making the response to insulin inconsistent.

At the same time, passive glucose movement and alternative pathways begin to play a larger role. Increased membrane permeability allows glucose to enter or leave cells outside of regulated transport mechanisms, reducing control over intracellular concentrations. This undermines the precision of glucose handling, as the system can no longer rely solely on transporter-mediated uptake to maintain balance.

The system compensates by increasing insulin output, attempting to overcome reduced sensitivity. Higher insulin levels increase the probability of receptor activation, but they do not restore the structural conditions required for efficient signaling. The underlying issue remains. Receptors are still misaligned, propagation is still incomplete, and transporter deployment is still impaired. The result is persistent dysregulation despite increased input.

Over time, accumulation of glucose and intermediates alters metabolic pathways, further stressing the system. Increased flux through alternative pathways generates byproducts that can modify proteins and lipids, reinforcing membrane instability. This creates a cycle where signaling failure leads to metabolic changes that further degrade the membrane conditions required for proper signaling.

Glucose dysregulation is therefore a failure of coordinated signaling at the membrane. The pathways exist and can be activated, but the structure required to execute them fully is compromised. Restoring control requires restoring the membrane environment so that receptor activation, signal propagation, and transporter deployment occur within a stable and organized framework, allowing glucose to be handled as a regulated input rather than a variable that the system cannot fully control.

Fat Oxidation and Mitochondrial Access

Fat oxidation is limited by whether fatty acids can be moved from their point of release to the mitochondrial matrix under controlled conditions. The pathway is sequential and boundary-dependent. Fatty acids must first be liberated, then transported through the cytosol, activated, and finally transferred across the mitochondrial membranes where oxidation occurs. Each step depends on membrane structure to maintain gradients, organize transport proteins, and preserve the conditions required for directional flow. When these conditions are stable, fatty acids are delivered efficiently to the mitochondria. When they are not, movement becomes fragmented, and access to oxidation pathways is reduced even if substrate is abundant.

Entry into the mitochondrial system is constrained by the outer and inner membranes. The outer membrane allows passage of activated fatty acids through specific channels, but the inner membrane imposes stricter control. Transfer across this boundary requires a coordinated system that converts fatty acids into forms that can be moved through dedicated transporters. This process depends on membrane integrity and the availability of transport proteins positioned within the correct lipid environment. If membrane composition alters transporter conformation or positioning, transfer slows or becomes inconsistent, limiting the rate at which fatty acids reach the matrix.

Activation and transport must remain coupled. Fatty acids are activated in the cytosol, forming intermediates that are then handed off to transport systems at the mitochondrial surface. If this handoff is delayed due to disrupted membrane organization, intermediates accumulate and are redirected into storage or alternative pathways. This reduces the proportion of fatty acids entering oxidation and increases reliance on other fuels. The system appears to have access to fat, but it cannot efficiently route that fat into the mitochondrial pathway.

Membrane composition influences this routing by affecting both transporter function and substrate partitioning. Fatty acids interact with membranes before entering transport pathways, and their distribution within the bilayer determines how accessible they are to activation enzymes and transport proteins. A membrane that supports organized domains can concentrate these substrates in regions where processing occurs efficiently. Disordered membranes disperse them, reducing the likelihood of coordinated activation and transfer.

Once inside the mitochondrion, oxidation depends on the inner membrane maintaining a stable gradient. If proton leakage increases or membrane structure is compromised, the rate of oxidation must rise to sustain ATP production. This increases demand for fatty acids, but if access to the matrix is already limited, the system cannot meet this demand efficiently. The result is a mismatch where oxidation capacity is stressed while substrate delivery remains constrained.

Hormonal signaling that regulates fat oxidation is also dependent on membrane state. Signals that promote fatty acid mobilization and mitochondrial uptake require coordinated receptor activation and downstream pathway engagement. When membrane structure is unstable, these signals are processed inconsistently, leading to periods where fatty acids are released but not effectively oxidized. This contributes to accumulation of intermediates and shifts in fuel utilization.

Electrical and ionic conditions influence mitochondrial access indirectly. Changes in membrane potential affect transporter activity and the coupling between transport and oxidation. Calcium flux, which can stimulate mitochondrial activity, becomes less controlled when membrane permeability increases, altering the rate at which oxidation pathways are engaged. These changes add variability to a system that depends on precise coordination between transport and energy production.

Fat oxidation therefore depends on a continuous structural pathway from membrane release to mitochondrial processing. Each boundary must maintain conditions that support controlled transfer and alignment of processes. When these conditions are intact, fatty acids move efficiently into oxidation. When they are not, the pathway fragments, and access to mitochondrial metabolism becomes limited despite the presence of available substrate.

Loss of Metabolic Flexibility

Metabolic flexibility depends on the system's ability to switch between fuel sources by coordinating transport, signaling, and mitochondrial processing within a stable membrane framework. This switching is not a simple preference shift. It requires synchronized changes in substrate entry, enzyme activity, and hormonal signaling so that one pathway ramps up as another downregulates. The membrane enforces this coordination by maintaining gradients, organizing receptors, and positioning transport systems. When these conditions drift, the system loses the ability to transition cleanly and becomes locked into inefficient or mismatched fuel use.

Fuel switching begins at the membrane with hormonal input. Signals such as insulin and glucagon must be translated into changes in transporter activity and enzyme regulation. This translation requires consistent receptor sensitivity and reliable propagation of signaling pathways. When membrane structure supports clustering and alignment, these signals produce coordinated adjustments in glucose and fat utilization. When structure is unstable, signaling becomes inconsistent. The system may attempt to switch fuels, but the response is incomplete or delayed, leading to overlap between pathways that should be mutually regulated.

Transport processes reflect this breakdown. Glucose and fatty acids enter cells through distinct mechanisms that rely on gradients and membrane organization. In a flexible system, these processes adjust dynamically based on demand. When membrane integrity is compromised, transport becomes less responsive. Glucose uptake may remain elevated when it should decline, or fatty acid entry may be limited when oxidation is required. The result is a mismatch between available substrates and metabolic pathways, forcing the system to operate under suboptimal conditions.

Mitochondrial function further constrains flexibility. Switching between fuels requires the mitochondria to adjust oxidation pathways while maintaining efficient ATP production. This depends on the inner membrane holding a stable gradient and supporting organized enzyme activity. Increased proton leakage or disrupted membrane organization reduces efficiency, making it harder for the system to adjust output in response to changing inputs. The mitochondria can still oxidize substrates, but they do so with less precision, limiting the system's ability to shift between fuels without accumulating intermediates.

Accumulation of intermediates signals incomplete transitions. When pathways do not downregulate or upregulate appropriately, partially processed substrates build up. These intermediates interfere with other metabolic processes, reinforcing the inability to switch cleanly. The system becomes constrained by its own byproducts, further reducing flexibility and increasing metabolic noise.

Electrical and ionic instability contributes to this rigidity. Fluctuating membrane potential alters enzyme activity and signaling thresholds, introducing variability into processes that require precise timing. Calcium flux, which influences both metabolic enzymes and mitochondrial activity, becomes less controlled, further disrupting coordination between pathways. These changes prevent the system from aligning multiple processes during a fuel transition.

Over time, repeated failure to switch fuels reinforces structural drift. Persistent reliance on one pathway alters membrane composition and signaling patterns, making alternative pathways less accessible. This creates a feedback loop where reduced flexibility leads to further structural changes that deepen the constraint. The system becomes biased toward a limited range of metabolic states, losing the ability to respond to varying demands.

Loss of metabolic flexibility is therefore a structural limitation expressed through metabolic behavior. The pathways for switching fuels remain present, but the membrane no longer provides the conditions required to coordinate them. Restoring flexibility requires restoring the structural framework that allows signals, transport, and mitochondrial function to align, enabling the system to transition between fuels without fragmentation or accumulation of intermediates.

Chapter 9

Neurological Function and Lipid Integrity

Neurological function depends on membranes that can maintain precise electrical separation while allowing controlled, rapid signaling across highly organized structures. Neurons operate through voltage changes that travel along membranes and across synapses. These processes require tight control of ion gradients, stable receptor positioning, and consistent membrane properties along extended cellular structures. Lipid composition determines whether these conditions hold. When membrane integrity is maintained, signals propagate with speed and precision. When it is not, timing shifts, signal strength varies, and communication between cells becomes unreliable.

The neuronal membrane is specialized for electrical control. Ion channels embedded within the bilayer open and close in response to changes in voltage, allowing rapid shifts in charge that generate action potentials. These channels depend on the surrounding lipid environment to maintain their conformation and responsiveness. Packing density and domain organization influence how channels transition between states and how quickly they can respond to changes in voltage. If the membrane becomes more permeable or disordered, ion gradients weaken, and channel behavior becomes less predictable. This alters the shape and timing of electrical signals as they move along the neuron.

Signal propagation along axons depends on maintaining these conditions over distance. The membrane must preserve electrical potential and prevent leakage as signals travel. Myelin adds an additional structural layer, increasing resistance to ion movement and allowing signals to move more efficiently. The composition of both the axonal membrane and myelin determines how well this insulation is maintained. Structural changes that increase permeability or disrupt lipid organization reduce conduction efficiency, requiring more energy to propagate signals and increasing variability in timing.

Synaptic transmission adds another level of dependence on membrane structure. Neurotransmitter release requires vesicles to fuse with the presynaptic membrane in a controlled manner. This process depends on membrane curvature, lipid composition, and the positioning of proteins that mediate fusion. When these conditions are stable, release occurs in a coordinated burst that matches the incoming signal. When membrane structure is altered, vesicle fusion becomes less efficient or less synchronized, reducing the precision of neurotransmitter release.

Receptor function at the postsynaptic membrane is similarly dependent on lipid organization. Receptors must be positioned within domains that allow them to interact with signaling proteins and respond to neurotransmitters. Changes in membrane composition alter receptor sensitivity, clustering, and coupling to downstream pathways. This affects how signals are received and processed, influencing everything from synaptic strength to overall network activity.

Electrical stability is reinforced by the ability of the membrane to maintain ion gradients. Sodium, potassium, and calcium gradients must be preserved to support repeated signaling. Increased permeability or disrupted transport processes weaken these gradients, requiring additional energy to restore them. This increases metabolic demand and reduces the efficiency of neuronal activity, especially under sustained signaling conditions.

Lipid composition also influences the production and regulation of signaling molecules within the nervous system. Fatty acids released from membranes can be converted into compounds that affect neuronal activity and local inflammation. The balance of these substrates determines the profile of signals generated during stress or injury, linking membrane composition to broader neurological responses.

Neurological function therefore reflects the state of membrane integrity across multiple levels. Electrical signaling, synaptic transmission, and metabolic support all depend on membranes that maintain structure and organization under continuous activity. When this structure is intact, the system operates with precision and efficiency. When it is compromised, variability increases, timing shifts, and communication between cells becomes less reliable because the physical framework required for controlled signaling is no longer maintained.

Synaptic Membranes and Signal Transmission

Signal transmission at the synapse depends on membranes that can organize vesicle fusion, control neurotransmitter release, and position receptors within a stable electrical environment. The presynaptic and postsynaptic membranes form a coupled system where timing, amplitude, and termination of the signal are determined by how well lipid structure supports these processes. The synapse does not rely on diffusion alone. It relies on tightly coordinated membrane events that convert an incoming electrical signal into a controlled chemical output and then back into an electrical response in the receiving cell.

At the presynaptic terminal, vesicle docking and fusion require specific membrane conditions. Vesicles must be brought into close proximity with the membrane, held in place, and then fused rapidly when an action potential arrives. This sequence depends on lipid composition that supports curvature and maintains the integrity of fusion sites. Proteins that mediate docking and fusion operate within this lipid environment, and their ability to function depends on how the membrane constrains and positions them. When packing and domain organization are stable, vesicles fuse in a synchronized manner, releasing neurotransmitter in a controlled pulse. When the membrane is disordered, docking becomes less stable, and fusion events lose coordination, producing variable release.

Calcium entry links electrical activity to vesicle fusion. Voltage-gated calcium channels open in response to membrane depolarization, allowing calcium to enter the presynaptic terminal. The local concentration of calcium near fusion sites determines how many vesicles release their contents. Membrane structure controls both the positioning of these channels and the diffusion of calcium once it enters. Stable domains keep channels and fusion machinery aligned, ensuring that calcium influx produces a rapid and localized response. Disruption of this organization spreads calcium more broadly or reduces its effective concentration at release sites, altering the amount and timing of neurotransmitter release.

The synaptic cleft defines the space through which neurotransmitters travel, but the postsynaptic membrane determines how that signal is received. Receptors must be positioned within domains that allow them to interact with scaffolding proteins and downstream signaling components. Lipid organization influences receptor clustering and stability, affecting how strongly and how quickly the postsynaptic cell responds. When receptors are properly organized, neurotransmitter binding produces a coordinated change in ion flow, generating a clear electrical signal. When organization is lost, receptor responses become less synchronized, reducing signal clarity.

Termination of synaptic signaling requires rapid clearance of neurotransmitters and resetting of receptor states. Transporters and enzymes responsible for this process depend on membrane integrity to function efficiently. The membrane must support the positioning and activity of these components so that neurotransmitters are removed quickly after release. If clearance is delayed due to structural disruption, signals persist longer than intended, overlapping with subsequent inputs and increasing noise within the system.

Electrical properties of the synaptic membranes integrate these processes. The ability to maintain ion gradients and respond to rapid changes in voltage determines how accurately signals are transmitted. Increased permeability or altered lipid composition changes how ions move across the membrane, affecting both the strength and timing of the postsynaptic response. This introduces variability into signal transmission, even if presynaptic release remains consistent.

Energy demand at the synapse is high, and mitochondrial support depends on local membrane conditions. If mitochondrial membranes are compromised, ATP production becomes less efficient, limiting the ability of the synapse to maintain ion gradients and recycle vesicles. This links synaptic performance directly to the structural state of membranes at multiple levels within the neuron.

Synaptic transmission therefore depends on membranes that can coordinate mechanical, chemical, and electrical processes within a confined space. Vesicle fusion, neurotransmitter release, receptor activation, and signal termination all rely on lipid organization and membrane integrity. When structure is intact, signals are transmitted with precision and timing that supports coherent network activity. When it is not, variability increases at each step, reducing the reliability of communication between neurons because the structural framework required for coordinated transmission has degraded.

Myelin Structure and Conduction Efficiency

Myelin establishes conduction efficiency by increasing membrane resistance and reducing capacitance along the axon, forcing current to travel longitudinally rather than dissipating across the membrane. The sheath is built as a multilayered lipid structure that compresses the bilayer into tightly packed lamellae. This packing excludes water, limits ion movement, and creates a high-resistance barrier around the axon. When this barrier is intact, depolarization generated at one node of Ranvier propagates rapidly to the next because current loss across the membrane is minimal. The signal advances in discrete steps, preserving amplitude and timing over distance.

Lipid composition determines whether this insulation holds under repeated activity. Myelin is enriched in cholesterol and saturated lipid species that support dense packing and mechanical stability. These lipids align to reduce free volume within the membrane, lowering permeability and maintaining consistent electrical properties. If packing loosens, even slightly, leakage increases. Current that should travel along the axon dissipates through the membrane, reducing the effective distance a depolarization can carry. The system compensates by requiring stronger or more frequent channel activation at the nodes, which increases energy demand and introduces variability in conduction speed.

The architecture of nodes and internodes depends on this lipid framework. Nodes of Ranvier concentrate voltage-gated sodium channels in narrow regions where the membrane is exposed. Between nodes, myelin insulates the axon and prevents ion exchange. This arrangement requires sharp boundaries between high-resistance myelinated segments and low-resistance nodal regions. Lipid organization maintains these boundaries by stabilizing the sheath and anchoring proteins that define nodal structure. When the lipid environment is altered, these boundaries blur. Channels may become mislocalized, and the distinction between node and internode weakens, disrupting the pattern of signal propagation.

Mechanical stability of myelin affects conduction over time. The sheath must maintain its structure despite constant electrical activity and physical stress. Lipid composition influences how well the layers adhere and resist deformation. Stable myelin maintains consistent spacing between layers, preserving its insulating properties. Structural drift introduces irregularities in thickness and packing, creating points where resistance drops and current leakage increases. These localized defects slow conduction and can distort signal timing as impulses pass through regions of differing electrical properties.

Ion gradient maintenance is indirectly dependent on myelin integrity. By reducing leakage, myelin lowers the amount of ion movement required to propagate a signal. This reduces the workload on ion pumps that restore gradients after each action potential. When myelin becomes less effective, more ions cross the membrane during propagation, increasing the demand for active transport to re-establish baseline conditions. This raises energy consumption and can limit the ability of neurons to sustain high-frequency signaling.

Conduction efficiency therefore reflects the ability of myelin to maintain a high-resistance, low-capacitance environment along the axon. The lipid structure of the sheath enforces this condition by limiting ion movement and preserving electrical separation. When this structure is intact, signals travel rapidly and consistently. When it is compromised, current dissipates, timing becomes irregular, and the energy cost of signaling increases because the membrane no longer enforces the constraints required for efficient propagation.

Neuroinflammation and Lipid Breakdown

Neuroinflammation begins when membrane structure is disrupted and lipid components are released into an environment that interprets them as damage signals. Neuronal and glial membranes are built to maintain separation, electrical stability, and controlled signaling. When that structure is compromised, the contents of the membrane shift from structural roles into signaling substrates. This transition is not neutral. Fatty acids and lipid fragments that were previously contained within organized bilayers become available for enzymatic conversion into inflammatory mediators, initiating a local response that is driven by the condition of the membrane itself.

Breakdown of membrane phospholipids exposes fatty acid chains that serve as inputs for signaling pathways. Enzymes activated by stress or damage cleave these lipids, releasing substrates that are rapidly converted into compounds that alter vascular tone, immune cell behavior, and neuronal activity. The rate and type of these signals depend on the composition of the membrane. A membrane enriched with certain fatty acids will generate a different signaling profile than one built from a different substrate pool. This means that inflammation is not a uniform response. It is shaped by the structural composition of the membranes undergoing breakdown.

The local environment amplifies this process. Microglia and astrocytes respond to changes in membrane integrity by increasing their activity, producing additional signaling molecules, and altering the behavior of surrounding cells. These responses are triggered by both direct detection of membrane fragments and by the signaling molecules derived from lipid breakdown. As activation increases, more enzymes are expressed that further process available lipids, sustaining and expanding the inflammatory response. The system becomes self-reinforcing as long as the supply of disrupted membrane material continues.

Membrane permeability changes during this process. As lipid organization degrades, ion gradients become harder to maintain, and cells experience shifts in calcium and sodium levels that further activate inflammatory pathways. Increased calcium entry stimulates enzymes that break down additional membrane components, linking electrical instability to structural degradation. This creates a loop where membrane damage leads to ionic disruption, which in turn accelerates further membrane breakdown.

Mitochondrial involvement intensifies the response. When mitochondrial membranes are compromised, reactive species production increases, and energy output becomes less efficient. This reduces the ability of cells to restore membrane integrity while simultaneously increasing the signals that drive inflammation. Mitochondrial lipid components can also become part of the signaling environment when released, further contributing to the perception of damage within the tissue.

Clearance and resolution depend on the system's ability to process and remove the products of lipid breakdown. Specialized pathways convert inflammatory signals into compounds that promote resolution and repair, but this requires that the signaling cascade proceed in an ordered sequence. If membrane damage persists or if the balance of lipid substrates favors continued activation, the transition to resolution is delayed. Signals overlap, and the inflammatory state remains active beyond its initial purpose.

Neuroinflammation therefore reflects the state of lipid structure within neural tissue. It is initiated by the release and conversion of membrane components, shaped by the composition of those membranes, and sustained by feedback between structural damage and cellular response.

When membranes maintain integrity, these pathways remain contained and controlled. When they break down, the resulting signals drive a response that continues as long as the structural disruption persists because the system is reacting directly to the loss of organized lipid architecture.

Cognitive Instability as Structural Inconsistency

Cognitive stability depends on neural networks that can maintain consistent signal timing, amplitude, and integration across distributed regions. This consistency is enforced at the level of membrane structure, where ion gradients, receptor positioning, and synaptic transmission are coordinated within a stable lipid environment. When this structural framework is intact, neuronal activity follows predictable patterns. Signals arrive with reliable timing, synaptic responses scale appropriately, and network-level processing produces coherent output. When the structure becomes inconsistent, variability emerges at each step, and cognition reflects that variability as instability in attention, memory, and decision-making.

Neurons rely on membranes to preserve electrical gradients that define their readiness to fire. Small changes in permeability alter how quickly these gradients dissipate and how easily they are restored. If membrane integrity fluctuates across regions or over time, neurons do not share a common baseline state. Some cells become more excitable, while others require stronger input to respond. This uneven excitability disrupts the synchronization required for coordinated network activity, leading to signals that are either amplified beyond their intended range or fail to propagate effectively.

Synaptic transmission amplifies these inconsistencies. Vesicle release, receptor activation, and neurotransmitter clearance must occur within narrow temporal windows to maintain signal fidelity. Structural variation in synaptic membranes changes how these processes unfold. Release may become irregular, receptor responses may vary in strength, and clearance may be delayed. These variations introduce noise into communication between neurons, reducing the precision with which information is encoded and transmitted.

Network-level effects emerge from the accumulation of these local inconsistencies. Cognitive processes depend on the integration of signals across multiple regions, each contributing specific components to the overall output. When timing and amplitude vary unpredictably, integration becomes less reliable. Signals that should align temporally may arrive out of phase, and those that should be suppressed may persist. This disrupts the formation of stable patterns of activity required for sustained attention and accurate recall.

Mitochondrial support influences this process by determining whether neurons can maintain their electrical and synaptic demands. Inconsistent membrane structure within mitochondria reduces the efficiency of energy production, limiting the availability of ATP needed to restore ion gradients and recycle synaptic components. Energy constraints do not shut down activity immediately but reduce the margin within which neurons can operate, making them more sensitive to structural variability.

Inflammatory signaling further contributes to instability. When membrane breakdown generates persistent signaling molecules, receptor activity and ion channel behavior are altered in ways that shift baseline excitability. These changes can occur unevenly across regions, adding another layer of variability to network function. The result is a system where both structural and signaling conditions fluctuate, preventing the establishment of stable cognitive states.

Cognitive instability therefore reflects a loss of structural consistency across the membranes that support neural function. The pathways for processing information remain present, but the conditions required for precise coordination are no longer maintained. As variability increases in electrical gradients, synaptic transmission, and energy availability, the system produces outputs that are less predictable and less stable because the underlying architecture no longer enforces uniform behavior across the network.

Chapter 10

Cardiovascular Function Reframed

Cardiovascular function is defined by the ability of blood vessels to maintain controlled flow, pressure distribution, and exchange across a continuously adapting network of boundaries. This system is often reduced to flow rates, pressure measurements, and circulating markers, but these outputs are downstream of structural conditions within the vessel wall. The endothelium and surrounding lipid membranes determine how signals are received, how the vessel responds to mechanical force, and how exchange with the bloodstream is regulated. When structure is stable, flow remains controlled and responsive. When it is not, the system shifts toward instability, where pressure, resistance, and signaling become inconsistent.

The vascular endothelium forms the primary interface between blood and tissue. This layer is not passive. It acts as a dynamic membrane system that senses shear stress, chemical signals, and changes in circulating substrates. Lipid composition within endothelial membranes determines how these signals are translated into functional responses such as dilation or constriction. Stable membrane domains support consistent receptor activity and coordinated signaling pathways. Disruption alters how these inputs are processed, leading to responses that are either exaggerated or insufficient relative to the demand.

Flow regulation depends on the ability of vessels to adjust diameter in response to local conditions. This adjustment requires rapid communication within the endothelial layer and between the endothelium and smooth muscle cells. Membrane integrity supports the propagation of these signals by maintaining receptor alignment and ion channel function. When structural consistency is lost, signal transmission becomes uneven, and changes in vessel diameter occur with less precision. This introduces variability into blood flow, even if overall pressure remains within a measurable range.

Exchange across the vascular boundary is also structurally controlled. Nutrients, gases, and signaling molecules must move between blood and tissue through regulated pathways. The permeability of this boundary depends on tight junctions and membrane organization. When lipid structure is maintained, exchange occurs selectively, allowing necessary substrates to pass while retaining structural integrity. Increased permeability due to membrane disruption allows uncontrolled movement of substances, altering the composition of both blood and surrounding tissue.

Mechanical forces act continuously on the vascular system. Shear stress from blood flow and pressure from circulation require vessels to maintain structural resilience. Lipid composition influences how membranes respond to these forces, affecting their ability to deform and recover without damage. Stable membranes distribute mechanical stress evenly, preserving function. Structural drift creates regions of weakness where stress is not managed effectively, leading to localized dysfunction.

Signal integration within the cardiovascular system depends on membrane-mediated processes. Hormonal signals, neural input, and local chemical cues all converge on the vessel wall. The endothelium processes these inputs and determines the appropriate response. When membrane structure supports organized signaling, these inputs are integrated into a coherent output. When it does not, signals compete or interfere with one another, leading to inconsistent regulation of vascular tone and flow.

Energy demand within vascular cells is tied to their ability to maintain gradients and respond to continuous stimuli. Mitochondrial efficiency supports these functions, and this efficiency depends on membrane integrity within the organelle. Reduced efficiency limits the capacity of vascular cells to sustain their regulatory roles, contributing to functional instability under stress.

Cardiovascular function therefore reflects the structural condition of the membranes that define the vessel wall. Flow, pressure, and exchange are emergent properties of this structure. When lipid organization is maintained, the system operates with controlled adaptability. When it is compromised, variability increases across multiple parameters because the boundaries that enforce coordinated behavior no longer maintain the conditions required for stable function.

Blood Vessels as Lipid-Regulated Systems

Blood vessels operate as boundary systems whose behavior is determined by the structure of the endothelial membrane and the lipid environment that supports it. Flow, pressure, and exchange are outputs that emerge from how this boundary senses mechanical force, organizes signaling inputs, and controls permeability. The vessel wall is not a rigid pipe. It is a responsive surface that adjusts continuously based on conditions within the blood and the surrounding tissue. Lipid composition within this surface determines whether these adjustments occur in a controlled and coordinated manner or drift into inconsistency.

The endothelium detects shear stress from flowing blood and converts it into biochemical signals that regulate vessel tone. This conversion depends on receptors and ion channels embedded within the membrane, positioned within lipid domains that support their function. When these domains are stable, shear stress produces predictable activation of pathways that lead to dilation or constriction. Changes in membrane composition alter how these forces are detected and processed. The same mechanical input can produce different outputs if receptor behavior shifts due to changes in the surrounding lipid environment.

Nitric oxide production is one of the primary outputs of endothelial signaling and depends on membrane conditions that support enzyme activation and substrate availability. The enzyme responsible for its production operates within a lipid context that determines its efficiency and responsiveness. Stable membranes allow consistent production in response to flow, promoting smooth adjustments in vessel diameter. Structural disruption alters this process, leading to reduced or irregular production and affecting the ability of vessels to regulate resistance.

Permeability of the vessel wall is governed by tight junctions and membrane organization. Lipid composition influences how closely cells adhere and how selectively substances can pass between them. When membranes maintain integrity, permeability remains controlled, allowing nutrients and gases to move as needed while preserving separation between blood and tissue. Structural changes increase permeability, allowing components to move across the boundary in an uncontrolled manner. This alters local environments and affects signaling within both compartments.

Communication between endothelial cells and smooth muscle cells depends on membrane-mediated signaling. Signals generated at the endothelial surface must be transmitted across the vessel wall to produce changes in contraction. This requires consistent receptor activity and ion movement, both of which depend on membrane structure. When lipid organization supports these processes, signals propagate effectively, and the vessel adjusts its diameter in alignment with demand. When it does not, communication becomes uneven, and regulation of tone loses precision.

Mechanical resilience of blood vessels is also tied to lipid structure. Membranes must withstand continuous deformation as pressure and flow fluctuate. Lipid composition determines how well membranes can absorb and distribute these forces without sustaining damage. Stable membranes maintain their properties under stress, preserving function. Structural drift creates variability in how different regions respond to the same force, leading to localized changes in behavior.

Energy production within vascular cells supports their ability to maintain gradients and respond to signaling inputs. This depends on mitochondrial membranes that sustain efficient ATP generation. When mitochondrial structure is intact, energy supply meets demand, allowing continuous regulation of vessel function. Reduced efficiency limits this capacity, making the system more sensitive to fluctuations in input.

Blood vessels therefore function as lipid-regulated systems where structure defines behavior. The endothelial membrane integrates mechanical, chemical, and electrical inputs and converts them into coordinated outputs that control flow and exchange. When lipid organization is maintained, this integration produces stable and adaptive function. When it is not, variability emerges across the system because the boundary that governs these processes no longer maintains consistent conditions.

Endothelial Membranes and Flow Dynamics

Flow dynamics emerge from how endothelial membranes sense shear, organize signaling, and control ion movement along the vessel wall. The surface facing the bloodstream is a continuous lipid boundary that converts mechanical force into coordinated biochemical output. Shear stress deforms the membrane and its attached structures, shifting the state of embedded receptors and channels. When lipid packing and domain organization are stable, this deformation produces a consistent signal that aligns enzyme activity, ion flux, and downstream responses. The vessel adjusts diameter in proportion to flow, maintaining distribution without oscillation. When membrane structure drifts, the same mechanical input produces variable signaling, and flow becomes uneven across segments that should behave as a single unit.

Mechanotransduction depends on spatial organization within the membrane. Receptors, adhesion complexes, and ion channels must be positioned within domains that preserve their coupling to cytoskeletal elements and signaling enzymes. Lipid composition determines whether these domains remain intact under continuous shear. Stable membranes keep these components aligned so that force applied at the surface is transmitted into a defined intracellular response. Disordered membranes uncouple this chain. Force is still applied, but it does not propagate through the same pathways with the same intensity, leading to inconsistent activation of downstream processes.

Ion movement at the endothelial surface shapes immediate responses to flow. Calcium entry follows mechanical stimulation and acts as a trigger for pathways that adjust vessel tone. The magnitude and localization of this calcium signal depend on membrane permeability and channel positioning. When structure supports tight control, calcium influx is rapid and localized, producing a precise response. Increased permeability or altered channel distribution spreads this signal or reduces its peak, weakening the coupling between shear detection and functional output.

Production of vasoactive mediators is tied directly to these membrane events. Enzymes responsible for generating signals that relax or constrict the vessel operate within specific lipid environments that influence their activity. When membranes maintain proper composition, these enzymes respond proportionally to shear, producing a stable relationship between flow and vessel diameter. Structural disruption alters enzyme responsiveness, shifting this relationship and introducing variability in how vessels react to the same conditions.

The continuity of the endothelial layer allows signals to propagate along the vessel. Cells communicate through junctions and membrane-associated pathways that transmit changes in state from one region to another. Lipid organization supports this propagation by maintaining consistent membrane properties across cells. When these properties vary, signal transmission becomes uneven, and coordination along the vessel is lost. Local segments may respond differently to the same flow, creating irregular patterns of resistance.

Mechanical stress interacts with membrane structure over time. Continuous exposure to shear requires the membrane to deform and recover without losing integrity. Lipid composition determines how well this cycle is sustained. Stable membranes maintain their properties under repeated stress, preserving consistent signaling. Structural drift leads to cumulative changes in how the membrane responds, altering sensitivity to shear and shifting flow dynamics even without changes in external conditions.

Energy availability influences the ability of endothelial cells to sustain these processes. Maintaining ion gradients, producing signaling molecules, and preserving membrane organization require continuous ATP supply. This depends on mitochondrial membranes that support efficient energy production. When energy production becomes less efficient, the system prioritizes basic maintenance over precise regulation, reducing the fidelity of flow control.

Flow dynamics therefore reflect the state of endothelial membranes as sensing and response surfaces. Mechanical input from blood movement is translated into biochemical and electrical outputs through lipid-dependent processes. When membrane structure is intact, this translation remains consistent, and flow is regulated smoothly across the vascular network. When structure is compromised, the link between force and response weakens, and flow becomes irregular because the membrane no longer enforces a stable relationship between input and output.

Cholesterol Transport as Repair Logistics

Cholesterol transport operates as a continuous repair system that moves structural material to sites where membranes require reinforcement or reconstruction. Cells do not treat cholesterol as excess cargo to be removed. They treat it as a component that must be redistributed to maintain membrane stability under changing conditions. Circulating lipoproteins act as transport vehicles that carry cholesterol through the bloodstream, delivering it to tissues where structural demand exceeds local supply. This movement is guided by signals that originate from membrane stress, damage, or increased mechanical load.

The process begins when cells alter their surface properties in response to structural need. Receptors at the membrane recognize circulating lipoproteins and initiate uptake based on these signals. This is not a passive accumulation. It is a targeted response that depends on membrane condition. When structural integrity is intact, uptake remains controlled. When membranes experience stress or disruption, receptor activity increases, directing more cholesterol into the cell. The system responds to structural demand rather than arbitrary concentration gradients.

Once internalized, cholesterol is routed toward membranes that require reinforcement. It integrates into the lipid bilayer, affecting packing density, permeability, and mechanical strength. Increased cholesterol content reduces free movement within the membrane, tightening structure and limiting ion leakage. This improves the ability of the membrane to maintain gradients and support embedded proteins. Redistribution within the cell ensures that areas under the greatest stress receive the highest concentration of structural material.

Transport in the opposite direction also reflects structural conditions. Cells release cholesterol when membrane composition shifts toward excess rigidity or when structural balance is restored. Lipoproteins that collect cholesterol from tissues carry it back through the circulation for reuse or processing. This bidirectional movement maintains equilibrium across the system, preventing localized accumulation while ensuring availability where needed.

The vascular system serves as the pathway for this logistics network, and endothelial membranes influence how lipoproteins interact with vessel walls. When endothelial structure is stable, transport occurs without significant retention. Lipoproteins pass through or interact transiently as part of normal exchange. Structural disruption alters this interaction. Changes in membrane permeability and receptor behavior can increase retention within the vessel wall, reflecting a local demand for repair material rather than a failure of transport.

Inflammatory signaling modifies this system by increasing the demand for cholesterol at sites of membrane damage. As lipid breakdown generates signals that recruit repair processes, lipoprotein uptake rises in affected regions. This links cholesterol transport directly to the state of membrane integrity. Persistent signaling maintains elevated transport, sustaining delivery as long as structural disruption continues.

Energy availability supports these logistics by enabling receptor function, vesicle trafficking, and intracellular redistribution. Efficient mitochondrial membranes provide the ATP required to maintain these processes.

Reduced energy supply limits the ability of cells to manage cholesterol movement effectively, slowing repair and altering distribution patterns.

Cholesterol transport therefore functions as a repair network that responds to structural conditions across tissues. Lipoproteins deliver and retrieve material based on membrane demand, maintaining balance through continuous redistribution. When membrane integrity is stable, this system operates quietly in the background. When structure is compromised, transport intensifies in affected areas because the system is responding to the need to restore the physical properties required for controlled cellular function.

Plaque as a Response, Not a Cause

Plaque formation begins as a localized response to disruption within the vascular boundary, not as an initiating event that drives dysfunction. The endothelium maintains separation between blood and tissue through a structured membrane that regulates permeability, signaling, and interaction with circulating particles. When this structure is compromised, the vessel wall shifts from a controlled interface to a reactive environment. Lipoproteins that normally transit through circulation begin to interact more directly with the vessel wall, not because they are inherently problematic, but because the boundary conditions that govern their movement have changed.

Disruption of endothelial membranes alters permeability and receptor behavior. This allows lipoproteins carrying cholesterol to enter or remain within the vessel wall in areas where structural integrity has weakened. Once present, these particles provide material that can be used for repair. Cholesterol integrates into local membranes, increasing packing density and reducing permeability in an attempt to stabilize the disrupted region. This accumulation reflects a functional response to structural need. The system directs available resources to reinforce areas where the boundary has failed to maintain its normal properties.

Inflammatory signaling accompanies this process because membrane disruption generates lipid-derived signals that recruit cellular activity. Immune cells enter the region and begin processing the accumulated material, interacting with both damaged membranes and retained lipoproteins. This activity is driven by the same signals that indicate structural damage. As long as these signals persist, the response continues, and the accumulation of material within the vessel wall increases.

Mechanical forces shape how this response develops. Regions of the vascular system that experience irregular flow or higher mechanical stress are more likely to exhibit structural disruption. These areas show increased interaction between lipoproteins and the vessel wall because the membrane must handle greater deformation and stress. The response in these regions reflects the need to stabilize a boundary that is under continuous strain.

Over time, repeated cycles of disruption and repair lead to the formation of a more permanent structure within the vessel wall. This structure contains lipids, cellular material, and extracellular components that together act as a reinforcement of the affected area. The persistence of this structure indicates that the underlying conditions driving the response have not been resolved. The system maintains the repair state because the boundary continues to experience stress or instability.

Energy availability influences the progression of this process. Cells involved in repair require ATP to maintain membrane integrity, process lipids, and manage signaling. Reduced mitochondrial efficiency limits the ability to complete repair cycles, prolonging the presence of intermediate states where accumulation continues without full resolution. This sustains the environment that supports plaque formation.

Plaque therefore represents a structural adaptation to ongoing disruption within the vessel wall. It forms as part of an attempt to restore stability in areas where the endothelial membrane has lost its ability to maintain controlled separation and signaling. The presence of plaque reflects the history of repeated repair responses rather than serving as the initial driver of dysfunction, because the system is responding directly to the loss of structural integrity at the vascular boundary.

Chapter 11

Immune System Precision

Immune function depends on the ability to distinguish between self and non-self, intact and damaged, signal and noise. This discrimination is not abstract. It is enforced through membrane structure, where receptors, co-receptors, and signaling complexes are organized into domains that determine how inputs are interpreted. Immune cells operate as boundary sensors that continuously sample their environment through membrane interactions. The precision of their response depends on whether these interactions occur within a stable lipid framework that preserves signal clarity. When structure is intact, responses are proportional and targeted. When it is not, detection becomes inconsistent and output loses specificity.

Recognition begins at the membrane with receptors that bind to molecular patterns. These receptors require precise positioning and clustering to initiate a response. Lipid organization determines whether receptors can assemble into functional complexes or remain dispersed and ineffective. In a stable membrane, receptor engagement produces a coordinated signal that propagates through defined pathways. Disruption alters receptor behavior, either lowering sensitivity so that relevant signals are missed or increasing baseline activation so that responses occur without appropriate triggers.

Signal amplification depends on the formation of microdomains that concentrate signaling components. These domains bring together enzymes, adaptor proteins, and ion channels that collectively determine the strength and duration of the response. Lipid composition influences the formation and stability of these domains, shaping how signals are processed. When domains are well-defined, amplification remains controlled and linked to the initiating event. When domain structure degrades, signaling becomes diffuse, and amplification can occur without proper regulation.

The immune response also depends on controlled activation thresholds. Cells must remain inactive under baseline conditions and respond rapidly when specific criteria are met. These thresholds are maintained through membrane-dependent processes that regulate receptor accessibility and downstream signaling. Structural drift shifts these thresholds, making cells either overly reactive or insufficiently responsive. This alters the balance between activation and tolerance, affecting how the system handles both external challenges and internal signals.

Communication between immune cells relies on membrane-mediated interactions. Cells exchange information through direct contact and through the release of signaling molecules that bind to receptors on neighboring cells. The efficiency of this communication depends on receptor function and membrane integrity across multiple cell types. When structure supports these processes, signals are transmitted with clarity, and coordinated responses emerge. When it does not, communication becomes fragmented, and responses lose coherence.

Energy availability constrains immune precision. Activation requires rapid changes in cell behavior, including proliferation, movement, and production of signaling molecules. These processes depend on mitochondrial function, which is itself dependent on membrane integrity. Reduced efficiency limits the ability of cells to sustain a controlled response, increasing variability in output.

Resolution of immune activity requires the system to transition from activation back to baseline. This process depends on signaling pathways that terminate responses and restore membrane conditions. Lipid-derived mediators play a role in this transition, linking membrane composition to the ability to complete the response cycle. If structural conditions do not support this transition, activation persists beyond its intended scope.

Immune system precision therefore reflects the structural state of the membranes that govern recognition, signaling, and communication. The system's ability to respond accurately depends on maintaining the conditions that allow signals to be interpreted without distortion. When membrane integrity is preserved, immune responses remain targeted and proportional. When it is compromised, variability increases, and the system loses the ability to distinguish effectively between different inputs because the structural framework required for precise discrimination is no longer maintained.

Membrane Recognition and Immune Discrimination

Immune discrimination is enforced at the membrane where recognition events are translated into activation or tolerance. Cells do not evaluate threats in isolation. They assess patterns presented at boundaries, comparing molecular structures against a baseline defined by intact membranes. This process depends on receptors that bind to specific features and on the lipid environment that determines how those receptors behave once engaged. The membrane defines whether a signal is interpreted as meaningful or ignored by controlling receptor positioning, clustering, and coupling to downstream pathways.

Recognition begins with contact between immune cell membranes and their targets. This contact creates a structured interface where receptors scan for specific molecular patterns. Successful recognition requires receptors to assemble into functional clusters that can generate a signal strong enough to cross activation thresholds. Lipid domains provide the platform for this assembly, concentrating receptors and associated proteins within defined regions. When these domains are stable, recognition produces a clear signal that can be amplified. When they are not, receptors remain dispersed, and binding events fail to generate sufficient output.

Discrimination between self and non-self depends on how these signals are integrated. Cells are constantly exposed to self-derived molecules that should not trigger activation. Membrane structure helps maintain this tolerance by controlling receptor accessibility and limiting spontaneous clustering. Stable membranes keep activation thresholds high enough to prevent unnecessary responses. Structural disruption lowers these thresholds by altering receptor distribution and baseline signaling activity, increasing the likelihood that weak or irrelevant signals will initiate a response.

Signal propagation following recognition requires coordinated activation of enzymes and ion channels. This coordination depends on the proximity of signaling components within the membrane. Lipid organization ensures that once a receptor is engaged, downstream elements are positioned to respond immediately. Disruption increases the distance between these components, weakening the connection between recognition and response. Signals may initiate but fail to propagate effectively, or they may propagate in an uncontrolled manner if inhibitory mechanisms are compromised.

Membrane composition also influences the presentation of signals from target cells. Cells under stress or damage alter their membrane properties, exposing or releasing components that indicate a change in state. Immune cells detect these changes through receptor interactions at the membrane interface. The clarity of this detection depends on both the target membrane and the immune cell membrane maintaining structure. If either side is altered, recognition becomes less precise, and discrimination between different states is reduced.

Termination of recognition signals is necessary to prevent continuous activation. This requires removal or internalization of engaged receptors and restoration of membrane conditions. Lipid structure supports these processes by enabling efficient receptor recycling and maintaining the integrity of domains that regulate signaling. When this structure is compromised, receptors remain active longer than intended or fail to reset properly, prolonging the response.

Membrane recognition and immune discrimination therefore depend on a stable lipid framework that governs how signals are detected, amplified, and resolved. The system distinguishes between inputs based on how effectively these processes are coordinated at the membrane. When structure is intact, recognition is precise and responses are appropriately scaled. When it is not, both sensitivity and specificity are altered, leading to responses that do not match the actual conditions because the membrane no longer enforces the constraints required for accurate interpretation.

Lipid Mediators in Immune Coordination

Immune coordination depends on the controlled conversion of membrane lipids into signaling molecules that direct the sequence, scale, and termination of the response. These mediators are not produced independently of structure. They originate from fatty acids embedded within membranes and are released when enzymatic activity acts on the bilayer. The composition of the membrane determines which substrates are available and therefore which signals can be generated. This creates a direct link between structural state and immune behavior, where the membrane defines the signaling capacity of the cell before any external trigger is applied.

Release of lipid mediators begins when membrane-bound fatty acids are cleaved in response to activation or damage. This process is tightly coupled to receptor signaling and ion changes that occur at the membrane. Once released, these fatty acids are rapidly converted into a range of compounds that influence immune cell recruitment, vascular behavior, and local cellular activity. The profile of these compounds depends on substrate availability. Different fatty acids lead to different signaling outputs, shaping how the response unfolds in both intensity and duration.

Coordination emerges from the timing of these signals. Early mediators promote recruitment and activation, increasing local activity to address the initiating condition. As the response progresses, the system must shift toward signals that reduce activation and promote resolution. This transition depends on the availability of substrates that support these later-stage mediators and on the enzymatic pathways that convert them. If membrane composition favors continued production of early-stage signals, the transition is delayed, and activation persists longer than intended.

Spatial control of these mediators is maintained by their local production and rapid turnover. They act near their site of origin, influencing neighboring cells through membrane interactions and receptor binding. Membrane structure affects both the rate of production and the ability of cells to respond to these signals. Stable lipid domains support consistent receptor function, allowing cells to interpret mediator signals accurately. Disrupted membranes alter receptor behavior, changing how signals are received and integrated.

Feedback mechanisms link mediator production to the state of the response. As immune activity increases, enzymes involved in lipid conversion become more active, amplifying signal generation. Resolution pathways must then counterbalance this by producing mediators that suppress further activation and initiate repair. This balance depends on maintaining the structural conditions that allow both sets of pathways to operate. If membrane integrity is compromised, feedback becomes skewed toward continued activation, and coordination breaks down.

Interaction between immune cells relies on shared interpretation of these lipid signals. Cells respond not only to direct contact but also to the local concentration of mediators that reflect the state of the tissue. Consistent membrane structure across cells ensures that these signals produce coordinated responses. Variability in membrane composition introduces differences in sensitivity and response, reducing synchronization within the immune network.

Energy supply supports the synthesis and turnover of lipid mediators. Mitochondrial efficiency influences the availability of cofactors and the capacity to sustain these processes. Reduced efficiency limits the ability to produce resolution signals and to terminate the response effectively, prolonging the presence of activating mediators.

Lipid mediators therefore act as the coordination layer of the immune system, translating membrane state into dynamic signaling that directs the response from initiation through resolution. Their production, action, and termination depend on the structural context of the membrane. When this context is stable, immune activity progresses through defined stages and resolves appropriately. When it is not, signaling becomes biased and prolonged because the membrane no longer provides the conditions required for balanced mediator generation and interpretation.

Failure of Resolution and Immune Overactivation

Resolution is a defined phase of the immune response that requires a shift in signaling from activation to termination and repair. This shift depends on membrane-derived substrates, enzyme activity, and receptor behavior aligning to suppress further recruitment and restore baseline conditions. When membrane structure supports this transition, activating signals decline as resolving mediators increase, and cellular activity returns to a controlled state. When structural conditions are altered, this transition does not occur cleanly. Activation persists because the system continues to generate and respond to signals that were meant to be temporary.

The failure begins at the level of substrate availability. Membranes supply the fatty acids required to produce both activating and resolving mediators. If composition favors substrates that drive continued activation, the system remains biased toward producing signals that recruit and stimulate immune cells. The pathways that generate resolving mediators depend on different substrates and enzymatic conditions. When these are limited or delayed, the balance shifts, and the system continues to operate in an activated state even after the initial trigger has diminished.

Enzymatic control of mediator production is also dependent on membrane conditions. Enzymes responsible for generating resolving signals must be properly positioned and activated within the lipid environment. Structural disruption alters their activity, reducing the efficiency of conversion from activating to resolving mediators. This prolongs the presence of signals that maintain immune cell recruitment and activation, preventing the system from transitioning into a phase of repair.

Receptor behavior reinforces this imbalance. Cells responding to inflammatory signals rely on membrane-bound receptors to detect changes in mediator concentration. When membrane structure is stable, these receptors adjust sensitivity as conditions change, allowing cells to respond to resolving signals and reduce activity. Structural drift alters receptor function, maintaining sensitivity to activating signals while reducing responsiveness to signals that should terminate the response. This creates a condition where the system continues to amplify activation despite the presence of signals that would normally suppress it.

Clearance mechanisms become less effective under these conditions. Removal of cellular debris, excess mediators, and damaged components is required to complete the response. These processes depend on membrane integrity to support phagocytosis, transport, and intracellular processing. When structure is compromised, clearance slows, leaving signals and materials in place that continue to stimulate immune activity. The environment remains in a state that resembles ongoing damage, even if the initial cause has been addressed.

Mitochondrial function influences the ability to complete resolution. Energy is required to support the synthesis of resolving mediators, the activity of clearance pathways, and the restoration of membrane structure. Reduced efficiency limits these processes, extending the duration of the response and increasing the likelihood that activation will persist.

Feedback loops sustain overactivation. Continued membrane disruption generates additional substrates for activating mediators, while persistent signaling maintains enzyme activity that produces them. Without effective resolution, these loops do not break. The system remains engaged in a state of incomplete response, where activation is maintained without progression toward repair.

Failure of resolution therefore reflects a breakdown in the structural and biochemical conditions required to terminate immune activity. The pathways for resolution remain present, but they cannot dominate the response because membrane composition, enzyme function, and receptor behavior no longer support the transition. Immune overactivation emerges from this imbalance, where activation persists not because of a continuous external threat, but because the system cannot complete the sequence required to return to baseline.

Autoimmunity as Boundary Confusion

Autoimmunity emerges when the immune system loses the ability to distinguish between intact self-structure and altered or misrepresented signals at the membrane boundary. This failure is not a random misfire. It reflects a breakdown in how membranes present identity and how immune cells interpret that presentation. Every cell communicates its status through the organization of its surface, where proteins, lipids, and associated molecules form a recognizable pattern. When this pattern is stable, immune cells interpret it as self and remain inactive. When structural conditions shift, that pattern changes, and the same cell can be interpreted as a target.

Membrane composition influences how identity is displayed. Proteins that signal self are embedded within a lipid environment that determines their orientation, clustering, and accessibility. Stable lipid domains maintain consistent presentation, allowing immune receptors to recognize these signals reliably. Structural disruption alters this presentation. Proteins may become misfolded, redistributed, or exposed in ways that do not match the expected pattern. Immune cells encountering these altered surfaces receive conflicting signals, increasing the likelihood of activation against self-tissue.

Recognition thresholds are affected by these changes. Immune cells rely on a balance between activating and inhibitory signals at the membrane interface. This balance is maintained through receptor interactions that depend on precise positioning within lipid domains. When membrane structure is intact, inhibitory signals counterbalance weak activation, preventing unnecessary responses. Structural drift shifts this balance by altering receptor distribution and signaling strength. Inhibitory signals may weaken while activating signals remain, lowering the threshold for response and increasing the probability of targeting self-components.

Inflammatory signaling reinforces boundary confusion. Membrane breakdown releases lipid-derived mediators that indicate damage, recruiting immune activity to the area. These signals do not distinguish between external and internal causes. They reflect the state of the membrane itself. As long as disruption persists, the environment signals ongoing damage. Immune cells respond accordingly, even if the source of disruption is intrinsic to the tissue rather than an external threat.

Antigen presentation adds another layer to this process. Cells process internal components and present fragments at their surface for immune evaluation. This process depends on membrane integrity to ensure that only appropriate fragments are displayed under controlled conditions. Structural instability alters this process, increasing the presentation of fragments that would normally remain contained. These fragments can be interpreted as foreign when presented in an altered context, contributing to immune activation against self-derived material.

Communication between immune cells propagates the response. Once activation begins, signaling molecules amplify and spread the reaction to other cells. If membrane conditions across the system are inconsistent, responses become uneven and difficult to regulate. Some regions may exhibit strong activation while others remain less affected, creating a patchwork of immune activity that lacks coordination.

Energy constraints limit the ability to restore boundary integrity. Repairing membranes, clearing signals, and re-establishing tolerance require sustained energy input. Reduced mitochondrial efficiency slows these processes, prolonging the state in which boundary signals remain ambiguous. This extends the period during which immune cells interpret self-structures as targets.

Autoimmunity therefore reflects a failure of boundary definition at the membrane level. The immune system responds to patterns that no longer align with its definition of intact self because structural conditions have altered how those patterns are presented. The response persists as long as this mismatch remains, driven by continuous signals that indicate disruption, even in the absence of an external threat, because the membrane no longer provides a clear and consistent representation of identity.

PART IV

DIETARY LIPIDS AS STRUCTURAL INPUTS

Chapter 12

What Dietary Fat Becomes

Dietary fat enters the body as a structural input that is broken down, transported, and reassembled into membranes, signaling molecules, and energy substrates. It does not remain in its original form, and it is not handled as a uniform fuel. The system deconstructs dietary lipids into components that can be selectively routed based on structural demand. Fatty acids, glycerol backbones, and associated molecules are absorbed, repackaged, and distributed through a transport network that delivers them to tissues where they are either incorporated into membranes or stored for later use. What dietary fat becomes is determined by how these components are allocated across structural and functional pathways.

Digestion reduces dietary fat into absorbable units that can cross the intestinal boundary. This process depends on bile and enzymes that interact with lipids within the lumen, converting them into forms that can enter intestinal cells. Once inside, these components are reassembled into transport structures that move through the lymphatic system and into circulation. This initial transformation separates intake from function. The fat that enters the bloodstream has already been reorganized into a form suitable for distribution, not direct use.

Transport through circulation directs these lipids to tissues based on demand. Cells take up fatty acids through mechanisms that depend on membrane structure and signaling state. Uptake is not uniform across all tissues. It reflects local conditions such as energy requirements, membrane turnover, and signaling needs. Once inside the cell, fatty acids are partitioned between storage, oxidation, and incorporation into structural components. This partitioning determines whether dietary fat contributes to immediate energy production or to longer-term changes in membrane composition.

Incorporation into membranes represents one of the primary fates of dietary fat. Fatty acids become part of phospholipids and other structural lipids that define membrane properties. The types of fatty acids available influence how membranes are built, affecting packing density, fluidity, and permeability. Over time, repeated incorporation shifts membrane composition, altering how cells behave. This is not a rapid process. It reflects cumulative input, where dietary fat gradually changes the structural characteristics of the system.

Fatty acids also serve as precursors for signaling molecules. When membranes are remodeled or broken down, these fatty acids can be converted into compounds that influence inflammation, vascular behavior, and cellular communication. The signaling profile that emerges depends on the composition of the membrane, linking dietary input to downstream signaling capacity. This connection is indirect but persistent, as membrane composition defines the pool of substrates available for conversion.

Storage provides another pathway for dietary fat. When intake exceeds immediate structural and energetic needs, fatty acids are stored in specialized cells. This storage is not inert. It represents a reservoir that can be mobilized when conditions change. The composition of stored fat reflects dietary patterns and can influence the types of fatty acids released during periods of increased demand, affecting both energy production and signaling.

Oxidation of fatty acids provides energy under conditions where they are directed toward mitochondrial pathways. This process depends on the ability of cells to transport fatty acids into mitochondria and maintain the conditions required for efficient oxidation. Structural factors influence this pathway by determining how easily fatty acids can be mobilized and delivered to the sites of oxidation.

Dietary fat therefore becomes part of an integrated system where structure, signaling, storage, and energy production are interconnected. The body converts intake into components that are distributed and reassembled based on need, with membrane composition acting as a central determinant of how these components are used. Over time, the characteristics of dietary fat shape the structural and functional behavior of the system because they define the material from which membranes and signaling pathways are built.

Digestion, Emulsification, and Transport

Dietary fat enters a system that cannot process it in bulk form. Lipids are hydrophobic and must be reorganized before they can cross aqueous environments and cellular boundaries. Digestion begins with mechanical dispersion and proceeds through chemical processes that reduce large lipid structures into smaller units that can be handled by enzymes. This transformation is not optional. Without it, fat remains inaccessible, passing through the system without integration. The process converts dense, aggregated material into dispersed particles that expose surface area, allowing enzymatic interaction to occur.

Emulsification establishes this dispersion. Bile-derived molecules interact with dietary fat, breaking it into smaller droplets and stabilizing them within the intestinal lumen. These molecules orient themselves at the interface between lipid and water, preventing droplets from merging back into larger masses. This increases the effective surface area and creates a condition where enzymes can access lipid substrates. The efficiency of this step determines how completely dietary fat can be processed. Poor emulsification leaves large droplets intact, limiting enzyme activity and reducing absorption.

Enzymatic digestion follows emulsification. Lipases act on the surface of these droplets, cleaving triglycerides into fatty acids and monoacylglycerols. This reaction is constrained by access. Enzymes cannot penetrate large lipid masses and depend on the interface created by emulsification. As digestion proceeds, products accumulate at the surface, and bile components maintain dispersion so that enzymes can continue to act. The rate of this process determines how much lipid is converted into absorbable units before it reaches the lower intestine.

Absorption requires these products to cross the intestinal membrane. Fatty acids and monoacylglycerols move toward the enterocyte surface, where they are taken up and reassembled into new lipid structures within the cell. This step depends on membrane properties that allow controlled entry while maintaining separation from the lumen. Once inside, these components are reorganized into transport particles that can move through the body without aggregating or disrupting aqueous environments.

Transport begins with the formation of these particles, which package lipids into a form compatible with circulation. They move through the lymphatic system before entering the bloodstream, bypassing immediate processing by the liver. This routing allows peripheral tissues to access dietary fat directly. The structure of these transport particles determines how they interact with cell membranes and how efficiently lipids can be delivered to tissues.

Distribution depends on recognition and uptake mechanisms at target cells. Enzymes at the surface of blood vessels act on circulating particles, releasing fatty acids that can be taken up by nearby cells. This process is localized, linking delivery to the metabolic state of specific tissues. Membrane structure influences both the activity of these enzymes and the ability of cells to absorb released fatty acids. When structure supports these interactions, delivery is efficient and targeted.

Residual components of transport particles are cleared and processed, completing the cycle. The system continuously breaks down, reassembles, and redistributes lipids, maintaining a flow of material that supports structural and energetic needs. Each step depends on maintaining interfaces between lipid and aqueous environments and on membrane conditions that allow controlled transfer across boundaries.

Digestion, emulsification, and transport therefore form a sequence that converts dietary fat into usable components and directs them to where they are needed. The process relies on creating and maintaining interfaces that allow lipids to be processed without losing structural control. When these steps function efficiently, dietary fat is integrated into the system as both structural material and energy substrate. When they do not, access is reduced, and downstream processes receive inconsistent input because the initial transformation and delivery of lipid components have been compromised.

Lipoproteins as Delivery Systems

Lipoproteins function as transport structures that move hydrophobic lipids through an aqueous environment while preserving control over where and how those lipids are delivered. They are not passive carriers drifting through circulation. They are organized particles built with a lipid core and a surface layer that allows interaction with cell membranes and enzymes. This structure enables them to carry triglycerides, cholesterol, and other lipids in a form that remains stable in blood while still being accessible for controlled transfer into tissues.

The architecture of a lipoprotein defines its behavior. The core contains hydrophobic lipids that cannot exist freely in circulation. Surrounding this core is a surface composed of phospholipids, cholesterol, and proteins that orient toward the aqueous environment. These surface components determine how the particle interacts with receptors, enzymes, and other structures within the vascular system. Different classes of lipoproteins vary in size, composition, and function, reflecting their role in either delivering lipids to tissues or redistributing them for reuse.

Delivery begins when lipoproteins encounter tissues that express the appropriate receptors or enzymatic activity. Enzymes located at the vascular surface act on circulating particles, releasing fatty acids from triglycerides. These fatty acids are then taken up by nearby cells. This process is spatially controlled. It occurs where metabolic demand or structural need signals for uptake. The lipoprotein does not decide where to deliver its contents. The receiving tissue defines the interaction through its membrane state and signaling profile.

Cholesterol transport operates through similar interactions but follows a more regulated pathway. Cells express receptors that bind to specific lipoproteins and internalize them, bringing cholesterol into the cell. This uptake is driven by structural demand. Membranes that require reinforcement or remodeling increase receptor activity, pulling in more cholesterol. The process is responsive rather than excessive. It reflects the condition of the cell rather than the absolute concentration of lipoproteins in circulation.

After delivering part of their contents, lipoproteins are remodeled. They shrink, change composition, and continue circulating, interacting with other tissues or returning to the liver for further processing. This continuous remodeling allows the same particle to participate in multiple delivery events, redistributing lipids across the system. The process maintains balance by ensuring that lipids are not confined to a single location but are available where needed.

The interaction between lipoproteins and the vascular wall depends on endothelial membrane integrity. When the endothelial surface is stable, lipoproteins move through circulation with minimal retention, engaging only where delivery is required. Structural disruption alters this interaction. Increased permeability or changes in receptor behavior can lead to prolonged contact between lipoproteins and the vessel wall, reflecting local demand for lipid material rather than a failure of the transport system itself.

Energy availability supports the processes that govern lipoprotein function. Receptor activity, particle remodeling, and intracellular processing all require ATP. Efficient mitochondrial membranes ensure that these processes occur continuously and with precision. Reduced energy supply limits the ability of cells to manage lipid delivery effectively, altering distribution patterns across tissues.

Lipoproteins therefore act as delivery systems that integrate transport with structural demand. Their design allows lipids to move through the bloodstream without disrupting the environment while remaining accessible for targeted uptake. The distribution of their contents is determined by membrane conditions at the tissue level, ensuring that lipids are directed toward areas that require them for structural maintenance, signaling, or energy production.

Incorporation into Membranes Over Time

Membrane composition is not fixed. It is continuously remodeled through the gradual incorporation of fatty acids derived from circulation, replacing existing components as membranes are repaired, expanded, or turned over. This process occurs at a pace defined by cellular activity and structural demand, not by immediate intake. Dietary fat enters the system, is distributed, and then becomes available as a substrate for membrane synthesis. Over time, repeated exposure to specific fatty acid profiles shifts the composition of membranes across tissues, altering their physical and functional properties in a cumulative manner.

Incorporation begins with the integration of fatty acids into phospholipids and other structural lipids within the cell. This requires enzymatic processes that assemble these components into the bilayer, positioning them according to the needs of the membrane. The selection of fatty acids is influenced by availability and by the requirements of the local membrane environment. Cells under mechanical or signaling stress may preferentially incorporate components that increase stability or adjust fluidity, aligning membrane properties with functional demands.

Turnover ensures that this incorporation is continuous. Membranes experience constant wear from mechanical forces, signaling events, and metabolic activity. Damaged or outdated components are removed and replaced with newly synthesized lipids. This replacement is not random. It reflects both the composition of available substrates and the conditions within the cell. Over time, this leads to a gradual shift where the characteristics of incoming fatty acids become embedded in the structure of the membrane.

The effects of this process are distributed across different cellular compartments. Plasma membranes, organelle membranes, and specialized structures such as synapses or mitochondrial membranes each incorporate lipids according to their specific requirements. Differences in composition between these compartments influence how each performs its function. Changes in input therefore produce distinct effects depending on where incorporation occurs, but the underlying mechanism remains the same.

Membrane properties emerge from this composition. Packing density, permeability, and the ability to support protein function depend on the types of fatty acids present. As incorporation proceeds over time, these properties adjust. This alters how receptors behave, how ions move across the membrane, and how signals are transmitted within the cell. These changes are not abrupt. They accumulate gradually, reflecting the ongoing replacement of membrane components.

Storage pools contribute to this process by providing a reservoir of fatty acids that can be mobilized when needed. The composition of these stores reflects prior intake and influences the types of fatty acids available for incorporation during periods of increased demand. This creates a link between past dietary patterns and current membrane structure, as stored lipids are drawn upon to support ongoing remodeling.

Energy availability determines the rate at which incorporation and turnover can occur. Synthesis of membrane components and their integration into existing structures require ATP and coordinated enzymatic activity. Efficient mitochondrial function supports this process, allowing membranes to be maintained and adapted as conditions change. Reduced energy supply slows turnover, prolonging the presence of existing components and limiting the system's ability to adjust composition.

Incorporation into membranes over time therefore represents a continuous restructuring of the body's boundaries based on available lipid inputs. The process integrates dietary fat into the architecture of cells, shaping membrane behavior across tissues. As new components replace old ones, the physical and functional characteristics of membranes shift, influencing how the system responds to mechanical forces, signaling inputs, and metabolic demands because the structure that governs these processes is being rebuilt incrementally.

Remodeling Cycles and Turnover

Membranes exist in a constant cycle of breakdown and reconstruction that maintains their functional state under continuous stress. This cycle is not occasional maintenance. It is a continuous process that replaces components as they are altered by mechanical force, signaling activity, and metabolic reactions. Lipids within the bilayer are subject to oxidation, enzymatic modification, and physical deformation, all of which change their behavior within the membrane. Turnover removes these altered components and replaces them with newly assembled lipids, preserving the structural conditions required for controlled permeability, signaling, and electrical stability.

Breakdown begins when membrane components are identified as no longer suitable for maintaining function. Enzymatic activity targets specific lipids, cleaving them from the bilayer and converting them into intermediates that can be reused or further processed. This removal is selective. It reflects local conditions such as stress, damage, or changes in signaling demand. The rate of breakdown increases when membranes are exposed to higher levels of mechanical or chemical stress, accelerating the need for replacement.

Reconstruction follows immediately through the synthesis and insertion of new lipids. Fatty acids from circulation or local stores are activated and assembled into phospholipids that match the requirements of the membrane. This assembly occurs within the cell and is directed toward membranes that require reinforcement or modification. The integration of new components must align with existing structure, maintaining continuity while adjusting composition. This requires coordinated activity between synthesis pathways and membrane insertion mechanisms.

Cycles of remodeling differ across cellular compartments. Membranes that experience rapid signaling or high mechanical load, such as neuronal synapses or vascular endothelium, undergo faster turnover than more stable structures. This variation reflects functional demand. Areas that rely on precise signaling or structural integrity must maintain tighter control over membrane composition, requiring more frequent replacement of components that drift from optimal conditions.

Turnover also interacts with signaling processes. Breakdown of membrane lipids generates intermediates that can act as signaling molecules, linking structural maintenance to cellular communication. This creates a feedback system where increased signaling activity can accelerate remodeling, and remodeling can influence the signaling environment. The balance between these processes determines whether the system maintains stability or shifts toward a state of persistent activation.

Storage pools provide material for reconstruction during periods of increased demand. Fatty acids stored in specialized cells or within the cell itself are mobilized and directed toward membrane synthesis when turnover rates rise. The composition of these stores influences the characteristics of the newly formed membrane, linking past inputs to current structural outcomes.

Energy supply constrains the entire cycle. Both breakdown and reconstruction require ATP to support enzymatic activity, transport, and synthesis. Efficient mitochondrial function ensures that turnover can proceed at a rate that matches demand. When energy availability is reduced, turnover slows, allowing altered or damaged components to persist within the membrane. This reduces structural consistency and affects downstream processes that depend on membrane integrity.

Remodeling cycles and turnover therefore maintain the structural framework that supports cellular function. By continuously replacing components, the system preserves the conditions required for controlled exchange, signaling, and energy production. When these cycles operate efficiently, membranes remain aligned with functional demand. When they are disrupted or slowed, structural drift accumulates, and the system begins to operate with components that no longer support optimal behavior because the process that enforces structural renewal is no longer keeping pace with the forces that degrade it.

Chapter 13

Saturated Fats and Structural Stability

Saturated fats function as structural inputs that influence how membranes maintain shape, resist deformation, and control permeability under continuous stress. Their defining feature is the absence of double bonds along the fatty acid chain, which allows them to pack tightly within the lipid bilayer. This packing reduces free movement between molecules, increasing membrane density and mechanical stability. When incorporated into membranes, saturated fatty acids contribute to a structure that resists disruption, preserves gradients, and maintains consistent behavior across varying conditions.

Membrane stability depends on the balance between rigidity and flexibility. Saturated fats shift this balance toward controlled rigidity by limiting the degree to which lipid chains can bend and move. This reduces the formation of gaps within the bilayer, decreasing permeability to ions and small molecules. The result is a membrane that holds electrical gradients more effectively and supports the function of embedded proteins that rely on stable conditions. Without sufficient structural support, membranes become more susceptible to deformation and leakage, altering how signals and substrates move across them.

Mechanical forces act continuously on cellular membranes, particularly in tissues exposed to pressure, flow, or repeated deformation. Saturated fats enhance the ability of membranes to withstand these forces by reinforcing the bilayer against distortion. This is especially relevant in systems where structural integrity directly influences function, such as vascular endothelium and neuronal membranes. A membrane enriched with saturated fatty acids distributes stress more evenly, reducing the likelihood of localized failure that can disrupt signaling or increase permeability.

Cholesterol interacts with saturated fats to further regulate membrane structure. The presence of saturated chains provides a framework within which cholesterol can integrate effectively, modulating membrane properties without destabilizing the bilayer. This interaction supports the formation of domains that organize receptors and signaling complexes. When saturated fats are present in appropriate proportions, cholesterol contributes to maintaining consistent membrane behavior. Without this structural context, cholesterol cannot exert the same stabilizing influence.

Saturated fats also influence how membranes respond to temperature and metabolic conditions. Their tight packing reduces the extent to which membranes become overly fluid at higher temperatures or under conditions that promote increased molecular movement. This maintains functional consistency across a range of environments, ensuring that membrane-dependent processes such as signaling and transport remain stable.

Incorporation of saturated fats into membranes occurs gradually through remodeling cycles. As new lipids replace existing components, the proportion of saturated fatty acids influences the long-term structural characteristics of the membrane. This cumulative effect means that dietary input contributes to membrane stability over time rather than producing immediate changes. The system integrates these inputs into its architecture, adjusting properties based on the available substrates.

Energy efficiency is indirectly supported by structural stability. Membranes that maintain tight control over permeability reduce the energy required to sustain ion gradients and support transport processes. This lowers the demand on mitochondrial function, allowing energy to be allocated more effectively across cellular activities. When membranes are less stable, increased leakage requires additional energy to restore conditions, reducing overall efficiency.

Saturated fats therefore contribute to the structural integrity of membranes by enhancing packing density, reducing permeability, and supporting consistent behavior under stress. Their role is defined by how they integrate into the lipid bilayer and interact with other components to maintain a stable boundary. This stability underlies the proper function of systems that depend on controlled gradients, organized signaling, and mechanical resilience because the membrane provides the physical framework through which these processes are executed.

Saturation and Membrane Rigidity

Membrane rigidity is determined by how tightly lipid molecules pack within the bilayer, and saturation directly controls this packing behavior. Saturated fatty acids have straight hydrocarbon chains that align closely with one another, minimizing space between adjacent molecules. This alignment reduces lateral movement within the membrane, increasing density and limiting deformation. As the proportion of saturated lipids rises, the bilayer becomes more ordered, and its physical resistance to bending, stretching, and compression increases.

This increased order reduces permeability. Tightly packed lipids create fewer transient gaps through which ions or small molecules can pass. Ion gradients depend on this containment. When membranes hold their structure, electrical potential can be maintained with minimal leakage, supporting processes such as signal transmission and active transport. As saturation decreases and packing loosens, permeability increases, and gradients dissipate more quickly, requiring greater energy input to restore them.

Rigidity also affects how proteins embedded within the membrane behave. Ion channels, receptors, and transporters operate within the constraints of the surrounding lipid environment. A more rigid membrane stabilizes the conformation of these proteins, allowing them to transition between states in a controlled manner. This supports consistent signaling and transport. When the membrane is less ordered, protein behavior becomes more variable, as the surrounding environment no longer constrains their movement with the same precision.

Mechanical stability emerges from this rigidity. Membranes are subjected to continuous forces, including shear stress, pressure, and cellular movement. Saturated lipids provide resistance to these forces by maintaining structural integrity under deformation. This reduces the likelihood of localized failure, where small disruptions in the bilayer can propagate into larger defects that alter function. A rigid membrane distributes stress more evenly, preserving its properties across different regions.

Cholesterol integrates into this environment and modulates rigidity further. In a membrane with sufficient saturated lipids, cholesterol fits between aligned chains, reinforcing packing and reducing fluidity without eliminating flexibility. This creates a state where the membrane remains stable but not brittle. If saturation is too low, cholesterol cannot stabilize the structure effectively, and if saturation is too high without modulation, the membrane can become excessively rigid, limiting necessary dynamic behavior.

Rigidity must therefore exist within a functional range. Membranes require enough order to maintain gradients and support protein function, but also enough flexibility to allow processes such as vesicle fusion, signaling, and transport. Saturated lipids establish the structural baseline, while other components adjust this baseline to meet functional demands. The balance between these elements determines how the membrane behaves under different conditions.

Over time, the level of saturation within membranes is shaped by the fatty acids available for incorporation. Remodeling cycles gradually shift composition, adjusting rigidity in response to input and demand. This process does not produce immediate changes but alters membrane properties through cumulative replacement of components.

Saturation and membrane rigidity therefore define the physical state of the bilayer, influencing permeability, protein behavior, and mechanical resilience. By controlling how tightly lipids pack, saturation sets the conditions under which cellular processes occur. When this structure is maintained within an appropriate range, membranes provide a stable yet responsive environment that supports consistent function across varying conditions.

Resistance to Oxidative Damage

Resistance to oxidative damage is determined by how vulnerable membrane lipids are to chemical attack and how effectively the system contains and repairs that damage when it occurs. Oxidation targets the double bonds within fatty acid chains. These sites are chemically reactive and can be altered by reactive species, initiating a chain reaction that propagates through adjacent lipids. Membranes with a higher proportion of unsaturated fatty acids present more of these reactive sites, increasing susceptibility. In contrast, saturated fatty acids lack double bonds and therefore provide fewer entry points for this process, reducing the likelihood that oxidative reactions will begin within the bilayer.

When oxidation is initiated, it alters the structure of affected lipids. The products of this reaction no longer fit within the membrane in the same way as intact fatty acids. This disrupts packing, increases permeability, and interferes with the behavior of embedded proteins. The initial event is localized, but if not contained, it spreads as adjacent lipids are affected. This propagation changes the physical properties of the membrane, leading to increased ion leakage and altered signaling. Resistance to oxidative damage therefore depends on both preventing initiation and limiting propagation.

Membrane composition influences both of these factors. A bilayer with tighter packing and fewer reactive sites reduces the probability that oxidative reactions will begin. Once initiated, dense packing also limits the spread of the reaction by restricting the movement of reactive intermediates. This containment reduces the scale of structural disruption and allows repair processes to address the affected area without widespread damage.

Antioxidant systems operate within this structural context. Lipid-soluble molecules positioned within the membrane can neutralize reactive species and interrupt propagation. Their effectiveness depends on distribution and accessibility, which are determined by membrane organization. When the bilayer maintains structure, these protective components remain properly positioned to intercept reactions as they occur. Disordered membranes reduce this effectiveness by altering distribution and allowing reactive species to move more freely.

Repair mechanisms follow containment. Damaged lipids are removed through enzymatic processes and replaced through remodeling cycles. This requires recognition of altered components and sufficient energy to support turnover. Efficient mitochondrial function supports these processes by providing the ATP necessary for enzymatic activity and synthesis. When energy supply is limited, damaged lipids persist longer within the membrane, extending the period during which structural properties are compromised.

The consequences of oxidative damage extend beyond the membrane itself. Increased permeability affects ion gradients, altering electrical and signaling conditions within the cell. Products of lipid oxidation can also act as signaling molecules, influencing inflammatory pathways and cellular responses. The extent of these effects depends on how well the initial damage is contained and repaired.

Resistance to oxidative damage therefore reflects a combination of structural composition and dynamic maintenance. Membranes that limit reactive sites, maintain tight packing, and support effective antioxidant and repair systems are less susceptible to disruption. When these conditions are met, oxidative events remain localized and are resolved without significant impact on function. When they are not, damage spreads and persists, altering membrane behavior and affecting the processes that depend on its integrity because the structural framework has been chemically modified and not adequately restored.

Thermal and Electrical Stability

Thermal and electrical stability emerge from how tightly the membrane controls movement at both the molecular and ionic level. Temperature increases kinetic energy within the bilayer, causing lipid chains to move more freely and increasing the probability of transient gaps forming between molecules. If the membrane lacks sufficient structural constraint, this increased motion leads to elevated permeability, loss of ion gradients, and disruption of protein function. Saturated fatty acids counter this effect by maintaining alignment and limiting chain movement even as temperature rises. Their straight structure reduces the degree of disorder that can develop under thermal stress, preserving the integrity of the bilayer across a wider range of conditions.

This thermal resistance directly influences electrical behavior. Membranes function as dielectric barriers that separate charge across a defined distance. The stability of this separation determines whether electrical gradients can be established and maintained. When thermal motion increases permeability, ions move more freely across the membrane, dissipating voltage differences and reducing the efficiency of processes that depend on controlled charge separation. A membrane with sufficient structural order resists this leakage, maintaining capacitance and allowing electrical signals to propagate with precision.

Electrical stability also depends on the uniformity of the membrane. Variations in lipid composition create regions with different conductive properties, which can distort signal transmission and alter how charge is distributed. Saturated lipids contribute to uniform packing, reducing heterogeneity in the bilayer and supporting consistent electrical behavior across its surface. This uniformity is critical in systems that rely on rapid and coordinated electrical changes, such as neuronal signaling and muscle contraction, where small disruptions in membrane properties can alter timing and amplitude of signals.

Cholesterol modulates both thermal and electrical stability by integrating between lipid molecules and adjusting how they respond to temperature changes. In the presence of saturated fatty acids, cholesterol restricts excessive movement at higher temperatures while preventing the membrane from becoming too rigid at lower temperatures. This creates a controlled range of fluidity that maintains both mechanical and electrical function. Without this interaction, membranes either become too permeable under heat or too rigid under cooling, each state impairing function in different ways.

Protein behavior is also tied to these properties. Ion channels and transporters depend on stable electrical gradients and consistent membrane thickness to operate correctly. Thermal instability alters the surrounding lipid environment, changing how these proteins shift between states. Electrical instability reduces the gradients that drive their activity. When both forms of stability are maintained, protein function remains predictable, allowing coordinated signaling and transport across the membrane.

Energy systems depend on this stability as well. Mitochondrial membranes rely on tightly controlled proton gradients to drive ATP production. Increased thermal motion or structural disorder allows protons to leak across the membrane, reducing the efficiency of energy conversion. Structural integrity limits this leakage, preserving the gradient and maintaining output. This links membrane composition directly to energy efficiency at the cellular level.

Thermal and electrical stability therefore arise from the same underlying structural conditions. A membrane that maintains tight packing, controlled fluidity, and uniform composition resists temperature-driven disorder and preserves charge separation. These properties allow gradients to persist, signals to propagate accurately, and energy systems to operate efficiently because the boundary itself continues to enforce the separation and containment required for these processes to occur.

Structural Necessity Under Stress

Stress exposes the membrane as a load-bearing structure rather than a passive boundary. Mechanical force, oxidative pressure, thermal fluctuation, and signaling intensity all converge on the bilayer at the same time. Each of these inputs increases movement within the membrane, distorts lipid packing, and challenges the ability of the system to maintain separation between internal and external environments. The requirement is not flexibility alone. The requirement is controlled resistance that preserves containment while allowing necessary function to continue. Saturated fatty acids contribute to this condition by maintaining alignment under force, limiting deformation, and preventing the formation of discontinuities that would allow uncontrolled exchange.

Mechanical stress acts first at the level of shape. Shear forces from blood flow, compression within tissues, and deformation during movement all push against the membrane. If lipid packing is loose, these forces create localized thinning and expansion, increasing the likelihood of transient defects. These defects allow ions and small molecules to cross in an unregulated manner, altering gradients and initiating downstream signaling that does not reflect controlled input. When saturated lipids are present in sufficient proportion, the bilayer distributes force across a larger area, reducing localized strain and maintaining thickness. The structure holds its geometry instead of collapsing into points of weakness.

Chemical stress follows through oxidation and reactive intermediates. Under these conditions, membranes with higher structural order limit both the initiation and spread of damage. Fewer reactive sites reduce the probability that oxidation begins, and tighter packing restricts the movement of reactive species once it does. This containment prevents the cascade from expanding across the bilayer. Without this constraint, damage propagates, altering multiple regions of the membrane at once and compromising function beyond the initial site of stress.

Thermal stress increases kinetic activity and amplifies both mechanical and chemical challenges. As temperature rises, lipid movement accelerates, and the likelihood of gap formation increases. A membrane that already lacks structural density cannot compensate for this increase in motion, leading to rapid loss of containment. Saturated lipids reduce the magnitude of this change by limiting how much additional movement occurs under heat. The membrane shifts, but within a constrained range that preserves function.

Signaling stress introduces a different form of load. High signaling demand requires repeated conformational changes in receptors, rapid cycling of ion channels, and continuous vesicle fusion and fission. These processes exert localized strain on the membrane and require a stable environment to operate correctly. Structural integrity ensures that these repeated events do not degrade the surrounding bilayer. When structure is insufficient, signaling becomes noisy. Receptors cluster irregularly, channels open and close unpredictably, and the system begins to interpret internal instability as external input.

Energy demand increases under all forms of stress. The cell must maintain gradients, repair damage, and support signaling at a higher rate. Structural stability reduces the energy required to perform these tasks. A membrane that holds its integrity minimizes leakage and limits the extent of repair needed, allowing energy to be directed toward function rather than compensation. When structure fails, energy is diverted toward restoring conditions that should have been maintained by the membrane itself.

Stress therefore reveals whether the membrane can enforce boundaries under load. Saturated fats contribute to this enforcement by stabilizing packing, reducing deformation, and limiting the spread of damage. This is not an enhancement layered onto function. It is a requirement for function to persist when conditions deviate from baseline. When structural integrity is maintained, the system continues to operate within defined parameters. When it is not, the boundary becomes inconsistent, and every process that depends on controlled separation begins to degrade because the physical framework that supports those processes is no longer stable under the forces acting upon it.

Chapter 14

Monounsaturated Fats and Adaptive Fluidity

Monounsaturated fats introduce controlled flexibility into membrane structure by inserting a single double bond into the fatty acid chain, creating a bend that disrupts tight packing without collapsing structural order. This geometric change prevents lipids from aligning as densely as saturated fatty acids, increasing lateral movement within the bilayer while still maintaining cohesion. The result is a membrane that can adjust its physical state in response to changing conditions without losing containment. This capacity for adjustment defines adaptive fluidity, where the membrane remains stable but capable of shifting its behavior as functional demands change.

Fluidity determines how quickly and efficiently components within the membrane can move. Receptors must cluster, channels must transition between states, and vesicles must fuse and separate from the bilayer. These processes require space and mobility within the lipid environment. Monounsaturated fatty acids provide this space by introducing slight irregularity into packing, allowing lipids to slide past one another without creating large gaps. This supports dynamic processes while preserving the continuity of the membrane, preventing the increase in permeability that would occur if structural order were lost entirely.

The balance between saturated and monounsaturated fats establishes a functional range of membrane behavior. Saturated lipids provide resistance to deformation and limit permeability, while monounsaturated lipids allow controlled movement and adaptation. Together, they create a membrane that can maintain gradients while still supporting dynamic processes. If monounsaturated content is too low, the membrane becomes overly rigid, restricting protein function and slowing processes that depend on movement. If too high, the membrane becomes less ordered, increasing permeability and reducing the ability to maintain controlled conditions.

Monounsaturated fats also influence how membranes respond to temperature. As thermal energy increases, the presence of kinks in fatty acid chains prevents excessive ordering that would otherwise restrict movement at lower temperatures, while still maintaining enough cohesion to prevent destabilization at higher temperatures. This creates a buffer against temperature-driven changes in membrane behavior, allowing function to remain consistent across a broader range of conditions.

Cholesterol interacts with monounsaturated fatty acids to refine this adaptive state. It positions itself between lipid molecules, reducing excessive movement when fluidity increases and preventing the membrane from becoming too rigid when fluidity decreases. In the presence of monounsaturated lipids, cholesterol helps maintain a controlled midpoint where the membrane can respond to changes without crossing into instability. This interaction allows the system to fine-tune its physical properties based on current demands.

Adaptive fluidity directly affects signaling. Receptor activation often depends on the ability to cluster within specific regions of the membrane, and this clustering requires mobility within the bilayer. Monounsaturated fats support this process by enabling lateral movement while maintaining the structural integrity needed for signal localization. This ensures that signals can be initiated and propagated without interference from excessive rigidity or disorder.

Energy systems also depend on this balance. Transport processes and gradient maintenance require membranes that can adjust without leaking. Monounsaturated fats allow minor structural shifts that accommodate changes in activity while preserving containment. This reduces the energy required to maintain conditions, as the membrane can adapt rather than resist all change or collapse under pressure.

Incorporation of monounsaturated fats occurs through the same remodeling cycles that govern overall membrane composition. Over time, their presence adjusts the functional properties of the membrane, shaping how it responds to mechanical, thermal, and signaling inputs. This gradual integration ensures that adaptive fluidity reflects sustained input rather than transient fluctuations.

Monounsaturated fats therefore provide the capacity for membranes to remain responsive without sacrificing stability. By introducing controlled disruption into lipid packing, they enable movement, support dynamic processes, and allow the membrane to adjust to changing conditions while maintaining its role as a boundary that enforces separation and control across the system.

Controlled Flexibility in Membranes

Controlled flexibility arises from the ability of the membrane to permit movement without losing structural continuity. The bilayer must allow lipids and proteins to shift position, change conformation, and reorganize locally while still maintaining a continuous barrier that preserves gradients and prevents uncontrolled exchange. This is achieved through the integration of monounsaturated fatty acids, whose single double bond introduces a bend in the hydrocarbon chain. This bend disrupts perfect alignment between neighboring lipids, creating space for lateral movement without generating the large defects that increase permeability.

This flexibility operates within defined limits. Lipids must move enough to support processes such as receptor clustering, vesicle fusion, and channel gating, but not so freely that the membrane becomes disordered. Monounsaturated fats provide this intermediate state by reducing packing density just enough to allow movement while maintaining sufficient cohesion to hold the bilayer intact. The membrane can deform locally to accommodate functional demands, then return to its baseline state once the demand subsides.

Protein function depends on this controlled environment. Embedded proteins rely on the surrounding lipid matrix to provide both support and mobility. If the membrane is too rigid, conformational changes required for activity are restricted, slowing signaling and transport. If too fluid, the lack of structural constraint alters how proteins shift between states, reducing precision. Controlled flexibility ensures that proteins operate within a consistent mechanical context, allowing predictable transitions and coordinated activity.

Flexibility also determines how membranes handle localized stress. During processes such as endocytosis or exocytosis, regions of the membrane must curve and reshape without fracturing. Monounsaturated lipids facilitate this by allowing lipids to rearrange under force, distributing strain across the bilayer. This prevents the formation of discontinuities while enabling the membrane to change shape as required.

The interaction with cholesterol further refines this flexibility. Cholesterol inserts between lipid molecules and adjusts how much movement is permitted. In areas where fluidity increases, it restricts excessive motion, maintaining cohesion. In areas where rigidity dominates, it disrupts tight packing enough to allow movement. This modulation keeps flexibility within a functional range, preventing extremes that would impair membrane behavior.

Electrical and transport functions are also influenced by this property. Ion channels and transporters depend on a stable yet adaptable membrane to maintain gradients while allowing controlled passage of substrates. Controlled flexibility ensures that these proteins can open, close, and cycle efficiently without introducing unintended leakage across the bilayer.

Over time, remodeling cycles adjust the level of flexibility by altering the proportion of monounsaturated lipids within the membrane. This gradual process aligns membrane behavior with sustained input and functional demand, rather than short-term fluctuations. The result is a membrane that reflects its environment while maintaining stability.

Controlled flexibility therefore defines how the membrane accommodates movement without compromising its role as a boundary. By allowing localized rearrangement while preserving overall structure, the bilayer supports dynamic processes and maintains the conditions required for signaling, transport, and energy production because the system can adjust without losing the containment that underlies all function.

Signal Modulation Through Fluid Balance

Signal modulation begins with how freely components within the membrane can move and organize in response to input. Receptors do not operate in isolation. They depend on lateral movement within the bilayer to cluster, separate, and interact with downstream partners. Fluid balance determines how quickly and precisely these arrangements form. When the membrane maintains controlled fluidity, receptors can assemble into functional groups at the right time and location, then disperse once signaling is complete. This movement is constrained enough to prevent random aggregation, but permissive enough to allow rapid reorganization in response to changing conditions.

Fluid balance influences the threshold required for signal initiation. In a membrane with appropriate mobility, receptors encounter one another with predictable frequency, allowing activation to occur only when sufficient input is present. If the membrane becomes too rigid, these encounters are limited, raising the threshold and slowing signal initiation. If too fluid, encounters become excessive and unstructured, lowering the threshold and increasing the likelihood of spontaneous or amplified signaling. The membrane therefore sets the baseline sensitivity of the system by controlling how often signaling components come into contact.

Signal amplification depends on the ability to concentrate activity within specific regions. Microdomains form when lipids and proteins co-localize, creating areas where signaling molecules are enriched. Controlled fluidity allows these domains to assemble without dispersing prematurely. Monounsaturated lipids enable the lateral movement required for this assembly, while surrounding structural elements prevent the domain from dissolving into the broader membrane. This balance allows signals to be strengthened locally without spreading indiscriminately across the cell.

Termination of signaling also relies on fluid balance. Once a signal has been transmitted, components must separate and return to a baseline state. If the membrane is too rigid, this separation is delayed, prolonging signaling beyond its intended duration. If too fluid, components may never remain associated long enough to complete the signal. Controlled fluidity allows both assembly and disassembly to occur with appropriate timing, ensuring that signals begin and end within defined windows.

Ion channel behavior is similarly affected. Channels depend on the surrounding lipid environment to maintain the structural conditions required for opening and closing. Fluid balance determines how easily these conformational changes occur and how stable each state remains. Excess rigidity restricts transitions, while excess fluidity destabilizes them. The membrane sets the conditions under which electrical signals are generated and propagated by controlling this balance.

Signal fidelity depends on consistency across the membrane. Variations in fluidity create regions with different signaling properties, introducing noise into the system. Controlled balance reduces these variations, ensuring that similar inputs produce similar outputs regardless of location. This uniformity allows coordinated responses across the cell, rather than fragmented or conflicting signals.

Metabolic state feeds into this system through remodeling cycles that adjust lipid composition over time. The proportion of monounsaturated lipids influences how fluid the membrane becomes, linking sustained input to signaling behavior. As composition shifts, the baseline sensitivity, amplification, and termination of signals shift with it, altering how the cell interprets and responds to its environment.

Signal modulation through fluid balance therefore reflects the physical state of the membrane rather than isolated biochemical pathways. By controlling movement within the bilayer, the membrane defines how signals are initiated, amplified, and resolved. When this balance is maintained, signaling remains precise and coordinated. When it drifts, the system becomes either unresponsive or excessively reactive because the structural conditions that govern interaction and timing are no longer aligned with functional demand.

Integration with Saturated Structures

Monounsaturated fats do not operate as independent modifiers of membrane behavior. Their function emerges only within the structural framework established by saturated lipids. Saturated fatty acids define baseline packing density, membrane thickness, and resistance to deformation. Monounsaturated fatty acids integrate into this framework by introducing localized disruption that allows movement without dissolving the overall structure. The relationship is not additive. It is interdependent. Without a stable saturated backbone, the flexibility introduced by monounsaturated lipids leads to loss of cohesion. Without monounsaturated input, the saturated framework becomes restrictive, limiting dynamic processes required for signaling and transport.

Integration occurs at the level of molecular packing. Saturated chains align tightly, forming regions of high order. Monounsaturated chains insert between these aligned lipids, creating controlled spacing that permits lateral movement. This spacing is not random. It is constrained by the surrounding saturated matrix, which prevents excessive displacement. The result is a membrane that maintains continuity while allowing localized rearrangement. Movement occurs within boundaries defined by structural density, preserving containment while enabling function.

Cholesterol stabilizes this integration by occupying the spaces created between lipid molecules and regulating how much movement is allowed. In regions where saturated lipids dominate, cholesterol prevents excessive rigidity by interrupting overly tight packing. In regions where monounsaturated lipids increase fluidity, it limits excessive motion by reinforcing interactions between neighboring molecules. This creates a dynamic equilibrium in which flexibility is continuously adjusted but never exceeds the limits required for structural integrity.

Protein function reflects this integrated state. Receptors and channels require both a stable platform and the ability to undergo conformational change. The saturated framework provides the mechanical support that maintains protein orientation and spacing. Monounsaturated lipids allow the surrounding environment to shift as proteins change shape during activation. Without this integration, proteins either become constrained within an inflexible matrix or lose the structural context required for precise operation.

Mechanical stress is distributed through this combined structure. Saturated lipids absorb and distribute force across the membrane, while monounsaturated lipids allow localized deformation that prevents fracture. This combination reduces the likelihood of structural failure under load. The membrane bends, stretches, and recovers without losing continuity because flexibility is embedded within a stable framework.

Electrical properties are also governed by this integration. The saturated backbone maintains low permeability, preserving ion gradients and electrical potential. Monounsaturated lipids allow the subtle adjustments required for channel activity and membrane deformation without introducing leakage. Together, they maintain the balance between insulation and responsiveness that defines electrical stability.

Remodeling cycles continuously adjust the ratio of saturated to monounsaturated lipids, refining this integration over time. Changes in input alter how these components are distributed within the membrane, shifting the balance between rigidity and flexibility. This process aligns membrane behavior with sustained conditions rather than transient fluctuations, ensuring that structure reflects ongoing demand.

Integration with saturated structures therefore defines how membranes achieve both stability and adaptability. Monounsaturated fats provide movement, but only within the constraints imposed by saturated lipids. This relationship allows the membrane to function as a controlled environment where dynamic processes occur without compromising the boundary that supports them, because flexibility is embedded within structure rather than existing in opposition to it.

Functional Tuning of Cellular Environments

Cellular function is not set by individual pathways acting in isolation. It is tuned through the physical state of the membrane, which defines how signals are received, how substrates move, and how energy is maintained. The ratio and distribution of saturated and monounsaturated lipids establish this state by determining packing density, lateral mobility, and permeability. These properties do not operate as abstract characteristics. They directly shape the behavior of proteins, gradients, and signaling networks embedded within the bilayer, creating an environment that either supports precise function or introduces variability.

Tuning begins with how the membrane sets baseline conditions. A structure with sufficient saturation maintains low permeability and stable gradients, providing a consistent internal environment. Monounsaturated lipids introduce controlled mobility, allowing the system to adjust without disrupting this baseline. The combination determines how sensitive the cell is to input. Increased rigidity raises the threshold for activation by limiting movement and interaction between signaling components. Increased fluidity lowers that threshold by allowing more frequent encounters. The membrane therefore defines whether the cell responds selectively or reacts to minimal input.

Receptor behavior is directly shaped by this environment. Activation depends on the ability to cluster and interact with downstream proteins. Controlled fluidity allows these clusters to form when needed, while structural density prevents uncontrolled aggregation. This balance determines signal strength and duration. A membrane that maintains proper tuning supports discrete, time-limited signaling events. When tuning is lost, signals either fail to initiate or persist beyond their intended duration, altering downstream processes.

Transport processes are similarly affected. Nutrient uptake, ion exchange, and waste removal all depend on proteins that operate within the membrane. These proteins require both structural support and the ability to transition between states. Saturated lipids maintain the conditions necessary for selective permeability, while monounsaturated lipids allow the conformational changes required for transport. The efficiency of these processes reflects how well the membrane maintains this balance, as excessive rigidity or fluidity disrupts the coordination required for controlled exchange.

Energy systems operate within the same constraints. Mitochondrial membranes rely on tight control of proton gradients, and any increase in permeability reduces efficiency. Structural density preserves these gradients, while controlled flexibility allows the membrane to adapt to changes in energy demand without introducing leakage. The ability to maintain output under varying conditions depends on how well the membrane sustains this tuned state.

Local variations within the membrane create specialized environments that support specific functions. Microdomains form where lipid composition and protein content differ from the surrounding bilayer, concentrating signaling or transport activity. Controlled tuning allows these domains to exist without destabilizing the broader membrane. Movement between domains remains regulated, ensuring that localized activity does not spread in an uncontrolled manner.

Remodeling cycles adjust this tuning over time. As lipids are replaced, the balance between saturated and monounsaturated components shifts, altering membrane behavior in response to sustained input. This process ensures that the cellular environment reflects long-term conditions rather than short-term fluctuations, aligning structure with functional demand.

Functional tuning of cellular environments therefore emerges from the integrated properties of the membrane. By controlling rigidity, mobility, and permeability, the bilayer defines how signals are processed, how materials are exchanged, and how energy is maintained. When this tuning is maintained, cellular processes operate with consistency and precision. When it drifts, variability increases, and the system begins to produce outputs that no longer match input because the structural conditions that govern behavior are no longer aligned with the demands placed upon them.

Chapter 15

Polyunsaturated Fats and Instability Risk

Polyunsaturated fats introduce multiple double bonds into the fatty acid chain, creating repeated bends that prevent close alignment within the membrane. Each double bond increases spacing between neighboring lipids, reducing packing density and increasing lateral movement. When incorporated into the bilayer, these structures expand the distance between molecules and weaken cohesive interactions that maintain membrane integrity. This does not immediately disrupt function, but it alters the physical conditions under which the membrane operates, shifting the system toward a more permissive and less constrained state.

Instability emerges from how this altered structure behaves under load. Reduced packing density increases permeability, allowing ions and small molecules to pass more easily through the membrane. This weakens gradients that depend on containment, forcing the cell to expend additional energy to maintain separation between compartments. At the same time, increased fluidity reduces the mechanical resistance of the membrane, making it more susceptible to deformation under pressure and shear forces. These changes do not occur in isolation. They compound, affecting signaling, transport, and energy systems simultaneously because all of these processes depend on controlled membrane behavior.

The presence of multiple double bonds also increases susceptibility to chemical modification. Each double bond represents a site where reactive species can initiate structural changes in the fatty acid chain. When these reactions occur, the resulting molecules no longer integrate into the membrane in a consistent way, further disrupting packing and increasing permeability. This creates a feedback loop in which structural instability promotes chemical damage, and chemical damage amplifies structural instability.

Signal behavior shifts within this environment. Increased fluidity allows receptors and signaling molecules to move more freely, lowering the threshold for interaction. This can lead to excessive or unregulated clustering, amplifying signals beyond their intended range. At the same time, the lack of structural constraint reduces the precision of these interactions, introducing variability into signaling outcomes. The membrane no longer enforces consistent conditions, and the system begins to produce outputs that do not reliably correspond to input.

Cholesterol attempts to compensate for this instability by inserting between lipid molecules and reducing excessive movement. However, its stabilizing capacity depends on the surrounding structure. In a membrane dominated by polyunsaturated lipids, the degree of disorder limits how effectively cholesterol can restore cohesion. The system remains more fluid and less controlled, even with regulatory input.

Mechanical stress exposes these limitations further. Under conditions of deformation, a membrane with reduced structural density cannot distribute force effectively. Localized strain leads to areas of thinning and increased permeability, allowing uncontrolled exchange across the bilayer. This compromises the boundary function of the membrane, affecting processes that depend on stable separation between internal and external environments.

Energy systems are directly impacted by this shift. Increased permeability leads to greater leakage of ions and protons, reducing the efficiency of gradient-dependent processes. Mitochondrial membranes, in particular, require tight control of proton gradients to sustain ATP production. Structural instability increases the energy required to maintain these gradients, reducing overall efficiency and placing additional demand on metabolic systems.

Remodeling cycles determine the extent to which polyunsaturated fats influence membrane behavior. As these lipids are incorporated over time, they alter the baseline properties of the bilayer, gradually shifting it toward increased fluidity and reduced structural constraint. This process reflects sustained input rather than immediate change, embedding these characteristics into the membrane architecture.

Polyunsaturated fats therefore act as structural modifiers that increase flexibility at the cost of stability. Their presence expands the range of motion within the membrane but reduces the system's ability to maintain controlled conditions under stress. When their proportion rises beyond what can be stabilized by saturated lipids and cholesterol, the membrane becomes more permeable, more chemically reactive, and less capable of enforcing the boundaries required for precise function because the structural framework has shifted toward a state that prioritizes movement over containment.

Structural Fragility of Multiple Double Bonds

Multiple double bonds introduce repeated disruptions along the fatty acid chain, preventing the linear alignment required for tight packing within the membrane. Each double bond creates a fixed bend that cannot straighten under normal physiological conditions. When several of these bends are present in a single molecule, the chain occupies more space and fails to integrate cleanly with neighboring lipids. This reduces cohesive interactions across the bilayer, increasing spacing between molecules and weakening the structural continuity that maintains membrane integrity.

This structural irregularity affects how force is distributed across the membrane. In a densely packed bilayer, mechanical stress is shared across aligned lipid chains, allowing the membrane to resist deformation. In a membrane enriched with polyunsaturated lipids, the lack of alignment creates points where force is not evenly transmitted. These points become areas of localized strain, where the membrane is more likely to thin, bend excessively, or form transient defects. These defects increase permeability and disrupt the controlled separation between compartments.

Chemical stability is also reduced. Each double bond represents a site where reactive species can interact with the fatty acid chain. With multiple double bonds present, the probability of these interactions increases. When a reaction occurs, it alters the structure of the lipid, creating products that no longer fit within the membrane in a consistent way. These altered molecules disrupt packing further, increasing the likelihood that adjacent lipids will also be affected. This propagation changes the physical properties of the membrane beyond the initial site of damage.

The combination of structural irregularity and chemical reactivity creates a condition where the membrane is more susceptible to both mechanical and chemical stress. Movement within the bilayer becomes less constrained, and the ability to maintain a continuous, stable boundary is reduced. Ion gradients depend on this continuity. As gaps form more readily, ions cross the membrane with less resistance, reducing electrical stability and increasing the energy required to maintain separation.

Protein behavior reflects these changes. Embedded proteins rely on a consistent lipid environment to maintain their structure and function. When the surrounding membrane becomes irregular and less stable, the mechanical context in which these proteins operate shifts. This alters how they transition between states, affecting signaling and transport processes that depend on precise conformational changes.

Cholesterol can partially mitigate these effects by inserting between lipid molecules and reducing excessive movement, but its ability to restore order is limited by the degree of disruption present. When multiple double bonds dominate the surrounding lipids, the overall structure remains less cohesive, and the stabilizing effect of cholesterol is reduced.

Structural fragility therefore arises from the cumulative impact of multiple bends within the fatty acid chain. These bends prevent tight packing, create points of mechanical weakness, and increase susceptibility to chemical modification. The membrane becomes less able to maintain its role as a controlled boundary, and the processes that depend on that boundary begin to operate under less stable conditions because the physical framework has been altered at the level of molecular structure.

Susceptibility to Oxidation

Oxidation targets the double bonds within fatty acid chains, and polyunsaturated lipids present multiple sites where this process can begin. Each double bond lowers the energy required for a reactive species to interact with the molecule, making initiation more likely under normal metabolic conditions. When a reactive species encounters one of these sites, it extracts an electron and creates a lipid radical. This altered molecule no longer behaves as a stable component of the membrane. Its structure shifts, and it becomes capable of reacting with neighboring lipids, extending the process beyond the initial point of contact.

Propagation follows initiation. The lipid radical reacts with adjacent fatty acids, particularly those that also contain double bonds, transferring the instability across the bilayer. This creates a chain reaction in which multiple lipids are converted into oxidized forms. These products do not align with intact lipids, disrupting packing and increasing spacing within the membrane. As this disruption spreads, permeability rises and the membrane loses its ability to maintain controlled separation between compartments.

The rate and extent of this process depend on both composition and organization. A membrane with a higher proportion of polyunsaturated lipids provides more reactive sites, increasing the probability of initiation and the speed of propagation. Reduced packing density allows reactive intermediates to move more freely, facilitating the spread of damage. In contrast, a more ordered membrane restricts movement and limits the reach of these reactions, containing them to smaller regions.

Oxidative products alter membrane behavior beyond structural disruption. They change how embedded proteins interact with the bilayer, affecting receptor activity, ion channel function, and transport processes. These changes are not uniform. They vary depending on the location and extent of oxidation, introducing variability into systems that rely on consistent conditions. Signaling pathways become less predictable as the physical environment shifts in response to chemical modification.

Repair mechanisms attempt to remove oxidized lipids and replace them through remodeling cycles. Enzymes identify altered molecules and extract them from the membrane, directing them toward processing pathways. New lipids are then synthesized and inserted to restore structure. This process requires energy and depends on the availability of suitable replacement components. When the rate of oxidation exceeds the rate of repair, damaged lipids accumulate, and structural disruption persists.

Antioxidant systems operate within the membrane to interrupt propagation. Lipid-soluble molecules can neutralize reactive species and stabilize radicals before they spread. Their effectiveness depends on distribution within the bilayer and the degree of structural organization. In a more disordered membrane, these systems are less able to contain reactions, allowing damage to extend further.

Susceptibility to oxidation therefore reflects both the number of reactive sites and the structural context in which they exist. Polyunsaturated lipids increase the likelihood that oxidation will begin and propagate, altering membrane composition and behavior. When this process is not contained and resolved efficiently, the membrane loses consistency, and the systems that depend on it operate under conditions that no longer support stable function because the lipid environment has been chemically modified and not fully restored.

Signal Amplification vs Signal Distortion

Signal amplification and signal distortion emerge from the same physical property of the membrane: how easily components can move, cluster, and interact within the bilayer. Movement allows receptors and signaling molecules to concentrate, increasing local activity and strengthening output. At the same time, excessive movement removes the structural constraints that keep these interactions specific, allowing signals to spread beyond their intended boundaries. The difference between amplification and distortion is not the presence of movement itself, but whether that movement remains confined within a structured environment.

Amplification begins when receptors and associated proteins are able to assemble into localized groups. Controlled fluidity allows these components to migrate toward one another and form clusters that increase the probability of interaction. Once clustered, signaling cascades proceed more efficiently because the necessary components are already in proximity. This reduces the time required for activation and increases the strength of the response relative to the initial input. The membrane acts as a platform that concentrates activity, allowing small signals to produce meaningful outputs.

This process depends on structural boundaries. Clusters must form within defined regions and remain stable long enough to complete the signaling sequence. Saturated lipids and cholesterol provide the framework that limits how far components can move and how long clusters persist. Within this framework, monounsaturated lipids allow the mobility required for assembly. When this balance is maintained, amplification remains localized and proportional to input.

Distortion occurs when this balance shifts toward excessive fluidity. Increased movement allows signaling components to interact more frequently but without the constraints that define where and when those interactions should occur. Receptors cluster unpredictably, signals spread across larger areas of the membrane, and the system begins to generate outputs that are not directly tied to specific inputs. The signal is no longer amplified in a controlled way. It is expanded beyond its intended scope.

This distortion affects both timing and intensity. Signals may initiate prematurely because components encounter one another too easily, lowering the activation threshold. Once initiated, they may persist longer than intended because clusters do not disassemble efficiently. The result is a loss of temporal control, where signals overlap or continue beyond the conditions that triggered them. This reduces the ability of the system to distinguish between different inputs.

Electrical signaling is also influenced by this shift. Ion channels depend on precise structural conditions to open and close in response to specific stimuli. Excessive fluidity alters these conditions, affecting how channels transition between states and how long they remain active. This introduces variability into electrical signals, affecting propagation and coordination across cells.

The products of lipid oxidation further contribute to distortion. Altered lipids disrupt packing and create regions with inconsistent properties, increasing variability across the membrane. These regions behave differently from surrounding areas, creating uneven signaling environments that amplify some signals while suppressing others. The membrane loses uniformity, and signaling becomes dependent on local structural conditions rather than consistent global properties.

Amplification therefore represents controlled concentration of activity within a stable framework, while distortion represents the loss of that framework, allowing activity to spread and persist without constraint. Both arise from the same underlying mechanism of movement within the membrane, but their outcomes diverge based on whether that movement is contained by sufficient structural organization. When the membrane maintains this organization, signals are strengthened without losing specificity. When it does not, the system produces outputs that no longer correspond accurately to input because the structural conditions that enforce precision have been disrupted.

When and Where They Are Appropriate

Polyunsaturated fats are not uniformly destabilizing or uniformly beneficial. Their appropriateness is determined by where they are placed within the system and what functional demand exists in that location. The same structural properties that increase fluidity and susceptibility to oxidation also enable rapid signaling, deformation, and responsiveness when those properties are required and properly contained. The question is not whether they should exist, but where their characteristics align with the demands placed on the membrane.

High-turnover signaling environments represent one of the primary contexts where polyunsaturated lipids are functionally appropriate. In membranes where rapid receptor movement, vesicle cycling, and signal propagation occur, increased fluidity allows components to reorganize quickly. This is relevant in synaptic regions, immune cell interfaces, and other areas where transient, high-frequency signaling is required. In these locations, the system compensates for structural fragility through increased turnover and localized control mechanisms that replace damaged components and limit the spread of instability.

Localized signaling domains provide another context. Polyunsaturated fats can be concentrated within specific microdomains where their mobility supports signal initiation and amplification. These domains are not the entire membrane. They are constrained regions within a broader structural framework dominated by more stable lipids. The surrounding structure limits how far the increased fluidity extends, allowing the system to benefit from rapid signaling without compromising global membrane integrity. This compartmentalization is critical. Without it, the same properties that enable signaling would introduce instability across the entire bilayer.

Precursor roles in signaling pathways also define appropriate placement. Polyunsaturated fatty acids serve as substrates for the generation of signaling molecules. Their presence within membranes allows rapid release and conversion when needed. This function requires accessibility rather than structural dominance. The membrane must contain enough of these lipids to supply signaling pathways without allowing them to define the overall physical state of the bilayer. This balance ensures availability without sacrificing stability.

Situations requiring rapid structural remodeling can also justify increased polyunsaturated content. During processes such as cell division, migration, or immune activation, membranes undergo significant deformation and reorganization. Increased fluidity facilitates these changes, allowing the membrane to reshape without fracturing. These conditions are temporary and localized. Once the demand subsides, remodeling cycles adjust composition back toward a more stable baseline.

Appropriateness is therefore conditional on containment and turnover. Polyunsaturated lipids function within systems that can replace them quickly, limit their distribution, and buffer their effects through surrounding structural elements. When these conditions are met, their properties support specific functional demands without destabilizing the membrane as a whole.

When these conditions are not present, the same properties become liabilities. Widespread incorporation into membranes that require long-term stability increases permeability, susceptibility to damage, and variability in signaling. The membrane loses its ability to maintain consistent conditions, and processes that depend on controlled boundaries begin to degrade.

Polyunsaturated fats are therefore appropriate in contexts that demand rapid movement, localized signaling, and dynamic restructuring, provided that these contexts are constrained within a stable framework. Their role is not to define the membrane, but to support specific functions within it. When their distribution expands beyond these controlled environments, the balance shifts, and the structural conditions required for consistent function are no longer maintained because the system has replaced containment with unrestricted mobility.

Chapter 16

Omega-3 Integration and Resolution Capacity

Omega-3 fatty acids enter the membrane as structural components that alter how the system handles signaling, deformation, and termination of stress responses. Their defining feature is a series of double bonds positioned in a way that increases chain flexibility while also enabling specific biochemical transformations. When incorporated into phospholipids, these fatty acids change local packing behavior, increasing spacing and mobility within the bilayer. This effect resembles other polyunsaturated lipids, but omega-3 integration carries an additional consequence. It alters the types of signaling molecules that can be generated from the membrane itself, shifting how the system initiates and resolves responses.

Integration occurs through standard remodeling cycles, where existing lipids are replaced with those available from circulation. Omega-3 fatty acids become part of the bilayer over time, distributing unevenly based on functional demand. They are often enriched in regions that require rapid signaling and dynamic behavior, such as neural membranes and immune interfaces. Their presence in these areas reflects a requirement for both responsiveness and controlled termination of activity, rather than structural reinforcement alone.

The primary functional impact of omega-3 integration lies in how these lipids are converted into signaling molecules. When membrane phospholipids are cleaved during activation, omega-3 fatty acids serve as substrates for the production of mediators that guide the progression and termination of responses. These mediators influence local cellular behavior by altering receptor activity, ion channel function, and gene expression patterns. The key distinction is not simply the initiation of signaling, but the ability to bring that signaling to completion.

Resolution capacity refers to the system's ability to terminate an activated state and return to baseline. This requires coordinated processes that reduce signaling intensity, clear cellular debris, and restore structural conditions within the membrane. Omega-3–derived mediators contribute to this process by shifting cellular behavior away from continued activation and toward restoration. They influence how immune cells interact with their environment, how vascular systems respond to stress, and how signaling pathways are downregulated once their purpose has been fulfilled.

Membrane composition determines whether this transition can occur efficiently. When omega-3 fatty acids are present in sufficient proportion, the system has access to the substrates required for generating resolution signals. When they are limited, signaling may proceed through initiation phases without a corresponding capacity to terminate, leading to prolonged activation. This creates a state where responses persist beyond their functional necessity, increasing structural and metabolic load on the system.

Integration must remain balanced with structural requirements. The multiple double bonds in omega-3 fatty acids increase susceptibility to oxidation and reduce packing density, which can compromise membrane stability if present in excess. Their incorporation therefore depends on containment within a broader framework that includes saturated and monounsaturated lipids. This framework preserves structural integrity while allowing omega-3 lipids to perform their signaling role.

Spatial distribution further refines their function. Omega-3 fatty acids are often concentrated in specific regions where their conversion into signaling molecules is most relevant. This localization ensures that their effects remain targeted rather than global, allowing resolution processes to occur where needed without altering the entire membrane environment.

Energy and repair systems support this integration by maintaining turnover and replacing oxidized components. Efficient mitochondrial function provides the energy required for these processes, ensuring that omega-3–containing membranes can be maintained without accumulating damage. Antioxidant systems also play a role in limiting the extent of oxidative modification, preserving the functional properties of these lipids.

Omega-3 integration therefore links membrane composition to the system's ability to complete its responses. By providing substrates for signaling pathways that terminate activation, these fatty acids influence whether processes resolve or persist. Their role is defined by how they are incorporated, where they are distributed, and how they interact with the surrounding structural framework. When integrated within a stable membrane architecture, they support the transition from activation to resolution, allowing the system to return to baseline after stress. When this integration is unbalanced, the same properties that enable signaling can contribute to instability because the structural conditions required to contain and complete these processes are no longer maintained.

Structural Incorporation into Membranes

Incorporation into membranes is a controlled, stepwise process that converts circulating fatty acids into fixed components of cellular structure. Fatty acids do not enter the bilayer in a free state. They are first activated within the cell, bound to carrier molecules, and directed into phospholipid synthesis pathways that determine how they will be positioned within the membrane. This assembly process selects which fatty acids occupy specific positions on the phospholipid backbone, shaping how each molecule behaves once inserted into the bilayer.

Insertion into the membrane follows synthesis. Newly formed phospholipids are delivered to existing membranes and integrated into the bilayer, where they replace older or damaged components. This replacement is not uniform across the membrane. Regions with higher activity or greater stress undergo faster turnover, leading to localized differences in composition. Over time, these differences create functional variation within the membrane, aligning structure with demand.

Omega-3 fatty acids alter membrane structure through their geometry once incorporated. Multiple double bonds introduce flexibility along the chain, increasing spacing between adjacent lipids and allowing greater lateral movement. This changes local packing density and influences how the membrane responds to deformation, signaling, and transport activity. The effect is not isolated to individual molecules. As more omega-3–containing phospholipids accumulate, the collective behavior of the membrane shifts toward increased mobility and altered interaction between components.

Position within the phospholipid molecule matters. Omega-3 fatty acids are typically incorporated at specific positions that influence how they interact with neighboring lipids and proteins. This positioning affects membrane curvature, domain formation, and the accessibility of these fatty acids for enzymatic release during signaling events. The structure of the phospholipid therefore determines not only how the membrane behaves mechanically, but also how it participates in biochemical processes.

Remodeling cycles continuously adjust this composition. Enzymatic systems remove existing fatty acids and replace them with those available in the cellular environment. This allows the membrane to adapt over time, integrating new inputs and discarding components that no longer support optimal function. The rate of this process depends on metabolic activity, energy availability, and the level of stress experienced by the cell.

Incorporation also influences interactions with cholesterol and other lipids. Omega-3–containing phospholipids alter how tightly cholesterol can pack within the membrane, affecting overall fluidity and domain organization. These interactions shape the distribution of signaling platforms and the behavior of embedded proteins, linking structural incorporation to functional outcomes.

Energy availability constrains the entire process. Synthesis, transport, and insertion of new phospholipids require ATP and coordinated enzymatic activity. When energy supply is sufficient, turnover maintains membrane integrity and adapts composition to current conditions. When energy is limited, incorporation slows, and existing components remain in place longer, even if they are suboptimal.

Structural incorporation into membranes therefore represents the mechanism by which external inputs become internal architecture. Through activation, synthesis, and targeted insertion, fatty acids are converted into components that define how the membrane behaves. Omega-3 fatty acids influence this behavior by altering packing, mobility, and interaction within the bilayer, embedding their effects into the structure over time rather than acting as transient modifiers of function.

Precursor Role for Resolving Mediators

Omega-3 fatty acids function as embedded substrates that can be released from the membrane and converted into signaling molecules that terminate active responses. Their role begins only after they are structurally incorporated into phospholipids. In this state, they are not circulating inputs. They are part of the membrane itself, positioned for rapid access when enzymatic systems are activated. When a cell transitions into an active state, specific enzymes cleave fatty acids from the phospholipid backbone, liberating omega-3 chains into the local environment. This release is tightly controlled and occurs at defined sites where signaling is required.

Once released, these fatty acids enter enzymatic pathways that convert them into mediators with specific functional effects. The structure of omega-3 molecules determines the types of mediators that can be produced. Multiple double bonds allow for transformations that generate compounds capable of altering cellular behavior in a directed way. These mediators do not initiate broad activation. They shift ongoing processes toward termination, reducing signaling intensity, promoting clearance of cellular debris, and restoring baseline conditions within the tissue.

The availability of these mediators depends entirely on prior incorporation. If omega-3 fatty acids are not present within the membrane, the system cannot produce them at the required time or location. Circulating fatty acids cannot substitute for this function because the timing of release must match the activation state of the cell. Structural incorporation ensures that the substrate is already in place, allowing immediate conversion when enzymes are engaged.

This process is spatially restricted. Release and conversion occur within localized regions of the membrane, often within defined microdomains where signaling activity is concentrated. This localization prevents widespread effects and ensures that resolution occurs where activation has taken place. The membrane therefore acts as both a storage site and a control surface, determining where and when these mediators are generated.

Competition between substrates influences which mediators are produced. Omega-6 and omega-3 fatty acids can both be released and processed by similar enzymatic systems, but they lead to different downstream effects. The relative proportion of these substrates within the membrane determines which pathway dominates at the moment of activation. This balance is not decided at the time of signaling. It is established through prior remodeling of membrane composition.

Termination of signaling requires more than a reduction in initial stimuli. It requires active processes that reverse the structural and biochemical changes associated with activation. Omega-3–derived mediators contribute to this by altering cellular interactions, reducing continued recruitment of signaling components, and supporting restoration of membrane conditions. These processes depend on coordinated activity across multiple cell types, but they originate from the availability of appropriate substrates within the membrane.

Turnover and repair systems maintain this capacity. As omega-3–containing lipids are used and removed, they must be replaced through remodeling cycles to preserve the ability to generate resolving mediators in future events. This creates a continuous dependency between membrane composition and functional capability.

The precursor role of omega-3 fatty acids therefore connects structure to the completion of biological responses. By existing within the membrane as accessible substrates, they enable the system to generate signals that bring activity to an end. When this capacity is present, responses proceed through initiation and resolution in sequence. When it is absent or reduced, activation can persist without an effective mechanism for termination because the structural components required to produce resolving signals are not available at the point where they are needed.

Time-Dependent Remodeling Effects

Membrane composition does not shift in response to a single input. It changes through continuous cycles of removal and replacement that operate over defined time scales. Each cycle extracts existing fatty acids from phospholipids and inserts new ones based on availability, energy status, and local demand. This process distributes change gradually across the membrane, altering structure in increments rather than discrete transitions. The functional state of the membrane at any moment reflects the cumulative result of these cycles, not the most recent input.

Turnover rates vary across tissues and compartments, creating different timelines for remodeling. Membranes exposed to high signaling activity or mechanical stress replace components more rapidly, allowing composition to adjust within shorter periods. More stable regions change more slowly, preserving existing structure over longer durations. This variation means that different parts of the system can exist at different stages of adaptation simultaneously, each reflecting its own balance between input and demand.

Omega-3 incorporation follows this same temporal pattern. As these fatty acids become available, they are inserted into membranes through repeated cycles, gradually increasing their proportion within specific regions. The effects on fluidity, signaling capacity, and resolution potential emerge as this proportion rises. There is no immediate shift in behavior. Instead, the membrane transitions through intermediate states, each with slightly altered properties. This progression determines how the system responds to activation over time.

Removal operates alongside incorporation. Fatty acids that have been oxidized, modified, or no longer support optimal function are selectively extracted and replaced. This prevents accumulation of components that would otherwise degrade membrane behavior. The efficiency of this removal process depends on enzymatic activity and energy availability. When turnover is sufficient, altered lipids are cleared before they can significantly affect structure. When it slows, these components persist, extending their influence on membrane properties.

Time dependence also governs how signaling capacity evolves. The balance between different fatty acid types within the membrane determines which mediators can be produced during activation. As composition shifts, the relative availability of substrates changes, altering the signaling profile of the cell. This change is not instantaneous. It follows the pace of remodeling, meaning that the system's ability to initiate or resolve responses adjusts gradually rather than abruptly.

Energy supply constrains the rate of these changes. Remodeling requires ATP for enzymatic activity, transport, and synthesis. When energy production is stable, turnover proceeds at a rate that maintains alignment between structure and demand. When energy is limited, both removal and incorporation slow, locking the membrane into its current state. This prolongs the presence of suboptimal components and delays adaptation to new inputs.

Time-dependent remodeling therefore defines how membrane structure evolves. Each cycle contributes a small adjustment, and the accumulation of these adjustments determines functional outcomes. The system does not respond to single events with immediate structural change. It integrates inputs over time, embedding them into the membrane through repeated replacement. As a result, the behavior of the cell reflects sustained conditions rather than transient fluctuations because the architecture that governs function is continuously updated through processes that operate on defined temporal scales.

Limits of Supplementation Without Structure

Supplementation introduces substrates into circulation, but it does not determine how those substrates are incorporated, distributed, or retained within the membrane. Structural outcomes depend on the state of the system that receives these inputs. Without an existing framework that supports controlled incorporation and turnover, added fatty acids remain loosely connected to function, moving through transport pathways without being embedded into stable architecture. The presence of a nutrient in circulation does not guarantee its integration into the structures that define cellular behavior.

Incorporation requires coordinated enzymatic activity, energy availability, and a membrane environment capable of accepting new components without destabilization. If the bilayer is already disordered, additional polyunsaturated inputs increase spacing and movement without restoring cohesion. This amplifies permeability and variability rather than correcting it. The system lacks the structural density required to contain the effects of these lipids, so their integration shifts the membrane further away from controlled behavior instead of toward it.

Turnover rate determines whether supplementation can influence structure. If removal and replacement cycles are active, new inputs gradually alter membrane composition over time. If turnover is impaired, existing components remain in place regardless of what is supplied. In this state, supplementation accumulates in circulation or storage pools without meaningfully changing the membrane. Structural conditions persist because the mechanism required to replace them is not operating at a sufficient rate.

Energy availability sets the upper limit on this process. Incorporation, remodeling, and repair all require ATP. When mitochondrial output is constrained, these processes slow, reducing the system's ability to integrate new substrates. Under these conditions, supplementation increases the burden on a system that cannot process it efficiently, leading to accumulation without functional integration.

Distribution also limits effectiveness. Fatty acids must be delivered to specific regions where they are needed, not simply present in the bloodstream. Without proper transport and targeting, inputs disperse unevenly, leading to localized changes that may not align with functional demand. This uneven distribution introduces variability across the membrane, affecting signaling and transport in inconsistent ways.

Structural context determines how supplemented fatty acids behave once incorporated. Omega-3 lipids, for example, require a surrounding framework of saturated and monounsaturated fats to maintain stability while enabling their signaling role. Without this framework, their presence increases susceptibility to oxidation and reduces packing density. The intended effect on resolution pathways is offset by increased instability at the level of the membrane itself.

Signaling capacity is also constrained by structure. The generation of mediators depends on the availability of substrates within the membrane and the organization of enzymatic systems that process them. Supplementation does not directly modify these systems. It only alters substrate availability. If the structural organization required for controlled release and conversion is not present, increased substrate does not translate into effective signaling.

The timing of supplementation relative to remodeling cycles further limits its impact. Inputs must be sustained long enough to be incorporated through repeated cycles. Short-term increases in availability do not produce immediate structural change because the membrane reflects cumulative replacement rather than transient exposure. This creates a delay between input and effect that cannot be bypassed by increasing dosage.

Supplementation therefore operates within the constraints of structure. It can supply the materials required for change, but it cannot impose that change on a system that lacks the capacity to integrate them. Structural integrity, energy availability, and active turnover determine whether inputs become part of the membrane or remain external to it. When these conditions are not met, supplementation fails to produce the intended outcome because the architecture required to translate input into function is not in place.

PART V

FAILURE PATTERNS IN MODERN SYSTEMS

Chapter 17

Industrial Lipids and Structural Breakdown

Industrial lipids enter the system as structurally altered inputs that do not align with the geometric and functional requirements of biological membranes. These molecules are often modified through processes that change the position, configuration, or stability of double bonds, creating fatty acid structures that differ from those naturally integrated into phospholipids. When incorporated into the bilayer, these altered geometries disrupt the packing patterns that membranes depend on to maintain cohesion, permeability control, and organized signaling.

The primary issue begins at the level of alignment. Membrane stability depends on predictable interactions between neighboring lipid chains. Industrial lipids introduce irregular shapes that do not conform to these interactions. Some configurations force chains into positions that create spacing inconsistent with surrounding lipids, while others produce rigid segments that fail to integrate into the dynamic movement of the bilayer. This mismatch alters local packing density, creating regions with inconsistent mechanical and electrical properties.

These disruptions affect how the membrane behaves under normal conditions. Increased irregularity leads to uneven permeability, where some regions allow greater ion movement than others. This variation distorts electrical gradients and introduces variability into signaling processes that depend on consistent membrane properties. The bilayer loses uniformity, and the system begins to operate with localized differences in behavior rather than a coordinated whole.

Protein function is directly influenced by these changes. Embedded proteins rely on a stable and predictable lipid environment to maintain their structure and transition between functional states. When the surrounding membrane contains irregular lipids, the mechanical context shifts. This alters how proteins fold, move, and interact with other components, reducing the precision of signaling and transport processes. The effect is not limited to a single pathway. It extends across systems that depend on membrane integrity.

Chemical stability is also compromised. Certain industrial lipid configurations are more susceptible to modification under physiological conditions, while others resist normal metabolic processing. This creates a condition where altered lipids either degrade into disruptive byproducts or persist within the membrane longer than intended. Both outcomes interfere with remodeling cycles that rely on the ability to remove and replace components efficiently.

Cholesterol interaction becomes less effective in this environment. Its ability to regulate fluidity and stabilize packing depends on the compatibility of surrounding lipids. When irregular structures dominate, cholesterol cannot position itself in a way that restores order. The membrane remains disorganized, and the regulatory capacity of cholesterol is reduced.

Mechanical stress amplifies these issues. Under deformation, regions containing incompatible lipids respond differently from surrounding areas, concentrating strain and increasing the likelihood of structural defects. These defects compromise the membrane's role as a boundary, allowing uncontrolled exchange and altering the conditions required for proper function.

Energy systems are indirectly affected through increased inefficiency. Variability in permeability leads to greater leakage of ions and protons, increasing the energy required to maintain gradients. This places additional demand on mitochondrial output, reducing overall efficiency and limiting the system's ability to support other processes.

Remodeling cycles attempt to correct these disruptions by removing incompatible lipids and replacing them with suitable components. The effectiveness of this process depends on turnover rate and the availability of appropriate substrates. If industrial lipids continue to be supplied, they are reintroduced into the membrane, preventing restoration of structural consistency.

Industrial lipids therefore contribute to structural breakdown by introducing components that do not integrate with the membrane's architecture. Their presence disrupts packing, alters permeability, and reduces the precision of signaling and transport. These effects accumulate over time, shifting the membrane away from a controlled and uniform state toward one characterized by variability and inefficiency because the structural inputs no longer match the requirements of the system they are attempting to support.

Seed Oils and High-PUFA Exposure

Seed oils deliver a concentrated load of polyunsaturated fatty acids that shifts membrane composition through repeated incorporation cycles. These inputs do not act at the level of immediate signaling. They enter circulation, are packaged into transport systems, and are gradually inserted into phospholipids as existing membrane components are replaced. Over time, this process increases the proportion of highly unsaturated chains within the bilayer, altering how lipids pack, how they move, and how they respond to stress. The effect is cumulative. Each remodeling cycle adds a small increment, and the accumulation of these increments defines the structural state of the membrane.

High-PUFA exposure changes packing density first. Multiple double bonds prevent close alignment between neighboring lipids, increasing spacing and reducing cohesive interactions. As these lipids accumulate, the membrane shifts toward a more permissive state with greater lateral movement and higher baseline permeability. This alters the containment properties of the bilayer, allowing ions and small molecules to pass more easily and increasing the energy required to maintain gradients. The system compensates by increasing transport activity, which raises metabolic demand without improving structural stability.

Chemical reactivity increases alongside these structural changes. Each additional double bond introduces a site that can undergo oxidation. As PUFA content rises, the number of potential initiation points for oxidative reactions increases, and the likelihood of propagation across the membrane expands. This creates conditions where localized chemical events can spread more easily, altering multiple regions of the bilayer and generating byproducts that further disrupt packing. The membrane becomes both more reactive and less capable of containing that reactivity.

Signal behavior shifts within this environment. Increased fluidity allows receptors and signaling molecules to encounter one another more frequently, lowering the threshold for activation. At the same time, reduced structural constraint weakens the boundaries that normally limit where these interactions occur. Signals become more diffuse, spreading beyond localized domains and persisting longer than intended. This introduces variability into signaling outcomes, as the membrane no longer enforces consistent conditions across its surface.

Cholesterol attempts to modulate these changes by inserting between lipid molecules and reducing excessive movement. However, its stabilizing capacity depends on the surrounding structure. When PUFA content dominates, the degree of disorder limits how effectively cholesterol can restore cohesion. The membrane remains more fluid and less controlled, even with regulatory input, because the underlying composition does not support tight packing.

Mechanical stability declines under these conditions. A membrane with reduced packing density cannot distribute force evenly, leading to localized strain during deformation. These regions are more prone to thinning and transient defects, increasing permeability and disrupting controlled exchange. This affects tissues exposed to continuous mechanical stress, where structural integrity is required to maintain function.

Remodeling cycles determine the persistence of these changes. As long as high-PUFA inputs continue, new lipids are incorporated at a rate that sustains or increases their proportion within the membrane. Removal of these components requires time and active turnover, meaning that the structural effects persist beyond the period of exposure. The membrane reflects long-term input rather than short-term variation.

High-PUFA exposure therefore alters membrane behavior through gradual but sustained changes in composition. Increased spacing, higher reactivity, and reduced structural constraint shift the bilayer toward a state that prioritizes movement over containment. This affects permeability, signaling precision, and energy efficiency because the structural conditions required for controlled function are progressively replaced with those that allow greater variability and less resistance to disruption.

Oxidized Fats and Membrane Damage

Oxidized fats enter or form within the membrane as structurally altered molecules that no longer behave like intact lipids. Oxidation changes the chemical configuration of fatty acid chains, introducing reactive groups, breaking segments, or creating cross-linked structures that disrupt how these molecules fit within the bilayer. When these altered lipids are present, they do not align with neighboring chains in a predictable way. This immediately affects packing density, increasing spacing in some regions while creating rigid, misaligned segments in others. The membrane becomes uneven at the molecular level, and this unevenness translates into functional instability.

Insertion of oxidized lipids alters permeability first. The bilayer depends on consistent alignment to limit the movement of ions and small molecules. When oxidized components create irregular gaps or distort surrounding lipids, these pathways open more easily. Ion gradients begin to dissipate as leakage increases, forcing the cell to expend additional energy to restore separation. This shift does not remain localized if oxidized lipids accumulate. It spreads across the membrane as more regions adopt similar irregular structure.

Propagation of damage follows through interaction with neighboring lipids. Oxidized molecules can initiate further reactions, altering adjacent fatty acids and extending structural disruption. This creates clusters of damaged lipids that behave differently from intact regions, increasing variability across the membrane. These clusters act as points of weakness where mechanical stress is concentrated and where permeability is elevated, further compromising the boundary function of the bilayer.

Protein behavior changes within this altered environment. Membrane proteins depend on a stable lipid matrix to maintain their structure and transition between functional states. When the surrounding lipids are irregular or chemically modified, the mechanical support they provide becomes inconsistent. This affects how proteins open, close, and interact with signaling partners, reducing the precision of processes that rely on coordinated activity.

Oxidized fats also generate secondary products that influence signaling pathways. These molecules can act as indicators of damage, triggering responses that alter cellular behavior. While this signaling can initiate repair processes, it also increases the overall activity within the system, adding to the structural and metabolic load. The membrane becomes both the source of damage and a participant in the response to that damage.

Removal and replacement are required to restore structure. Enzymatic systems identify oxidized lipids and extract them from the membrane, directing them toward processing pathways. New lipids are then synthesized and inserted to replace the damaged components. This process depends on sufficient energy and the availability of suitable substrates. If removal is slower than accumulation, oxidized lipids persist, extending their impact on membrane behavior.

Cholesterol and surrounding lipids cannot fully compensate for these disruptions. While they may stabilize adjacent regions, they cannot restore the original structure of altered molecules. The membrane remains heterogeneous, with areas that differ in permeability and mechanical properties.

Oxidized fats therefore act as structural defects within the bilayer. They disrupt packing, increase permeability, and alter protein function, creating conditions where the membrane can no longer enforce consistent boundaries. As these defects accumulate, the system operates with increasing variability and reduced efficiency because the physical framework that supports controlled exchange, signaling, and energy maintenance has been compromised at the molecular level.

Repeated Remodeling into Unstable Structures

Remodeling is intended to preserve membrane function by removing altered components and inserting new ones that restore structural integrity. When the input pool itself is unstable, this process no longer corrects the system. It reinforces the same instability with each cycle. Fatty acids are continuously exchanged within phospholipids, but if the available substrates are dominated by highly unsaturated or chemically modified lipids, every round of replacement shifts the membrane further toward a state of reduced packing density and increased reactivity. The process that normally maintains order becomes a mechanism that embeds disorder into the architecture.

Each remodeling cycle replaces only a fraction of the membrane at a time, but the cumulative effect is progressive. Newly inserted lipids alter local packing, which changes how adjacent lipids interact and how enzymes access the bilayer. This altered environment then influences the next cycle of replacement, favoring further incorporation of similar structures. Over time, the membrane transitions through intermediate states, each with slightly reduced cohesion and increased variability. There is no single point where instability begins. It emerges from the accumulation of small structural changes that are not corrected between cycles.

Instability compounds because newly incorporated lipids are more susceptible to modification. As these lipids undergo oxidation or mechanical distortion, they generate byproducts that interfere with surrounding structure and signaling. Remodeling removes some of these altered components, but if the replacement lipids share the same vulnerabilities, the system cannot resolve the underlying issue. The membrane remains in a continuous loop of incorporation, damage, and partial repair, without returning to a stable baseline.

This cycle affects how force and energy are managed. Reduced packing density increases permeability, allowing ions and protons to cross the membrane more easily. This increases the energy required to maintain gradients, placing additional demand on mitochondrial function. At the same time, mechanical stress is no longer distributed evenly across the bilayer. Regions with higher instability absorb more strain, leading to localized defects that further disrupt function. These defects alter both structural and electrical properties, amplifying variability across the membrane.

Signaling systems adapt to this changing environment. Increased fluidity and irregular packing alter how receptors cluster and how signals propagate. Activation thresholds shift, and termination becomes less precise. The system begins to operate with altered sensitivity and timing, not because signaling pathways have changed, but because the structural conditions that govern their behavior have drifted. Each remodeling cycle reinforces these conditions, embedding them more deeply into the membrane.

Cholesterol and remaining saturated lipids attempt to stabilize the structure, but their influence diminishes as the proportion of unstable lipids increases. Their ability to maintain order depends on sufficient surrounding alignment. As that alignment is lost, their regulatory effect becomes localized rather than global, leaving large regions of the membrane in a less controlled state.

Recovery requires a shift in both input and turnover. The system must not only remove unstable components but also replace them with lipids that restore packing density and reduce susceptibility to modification. This process takes time because each cycle replaces only a portion of the membrane. Until the input pool changes, remodeling continues to reinforce instability rather than resolve it.

Repeated remodeling into unstable structures therefore represents a failure of corrective processes under conditions where the available substrates do not support stability. The membrane is continuously rebuilt, but each reconstruction incorporates the same structural weaknesses, preventing the system from reestablishing a consistent and controlled environment because the inputs driving reconstruction do not match the requirements of the architecture they are meant to maintain.

System-Wide Signaling Distortion

When membrane structure drifts away from controlled packing and organized fluidity, signaling distortion does not remain localized. It propagates across systems because the same structural principles govern receptors, channels, and transporters in every tissue. The membrane sets the conditions under which signals are initiated, amplified, and terminated. When those conditions become inconsistent, the entire signaling network begins to operate with altered thresholds, timing, and intensity.

Distortion begins at the level of receptor interaction. Increased fluidity and irregular packing allow receptors to encounter one another more frequently, lowering the threshold required for activation. Signals initiate with less input and often without clear external triggers. At the same time, the lack of structural constraint allows these interactions to occur outside defined domains, spreading activation across larger areas of the membrane. What should remain a localized event becomes diffuse, reducing specificity and increasing background activity.

Propagation of signals changes as well. In a structured membrane, signaling complexes form within confined regions and transmit information through defined pathways. When structure is compromised, these complexes form and dissolve unpredictably. Signals can be amplified in one region and dissipated in another, depending on local membrane composition. This variability disrupts coordination between pathways, leading to outputs that are inconsistent even under similar conditions.

Termination becomes impaired. Controlled fluidity allows signaling components to separate once a response is complete. When the membrane is too fluid or irregular, these components remain associated longer than intended, prolonging activation. This extends signaling beyond its functional window, increasing the likelihood of overlapping or competing signals. The system loses temporal precision, and responses persist in the absence of appropriate input.

Electrical signaling is directly affected by these changes. Ion channels rely on stable membrane properties to open and close in response to specific stimuli. Increased permeability and structural variability alter the gradients that drive ion movement and change how channels transition between states. This introduces noise into electrical signals, affecting the timing and coordination of activity in excitable tissues.

Cross-system effects emerge because signaling pathways are interconnected. Changes in membrane structure in one tissue influence how signals are generated and interpreted in another. Hormonal signaling, immune responses, and metabolic regulation all depend on consistent membrane behavior. When distortion occurs, these systems receive and transmit signals that no longer reflect actual conditions, leading to mismatched responses across the body.

Feedback mechanisms amplify this distortion. Altered signaling can increase the production of reactive species, further modifying membrane lipids and reinforcing structural instability. This creates a loop where structural disruption leads to signaling changes, and signaling changes promote additional structural disruption. The system moves further away from controlled operation with each cycle.

Energy demand increases as the system attempts to compensate. Maintaining gradients, correcting signaling errors, and repairing structural damage all require additional ATP. This diverts resources from other processes and reduces overall efficiency. The system operates under increased load while producing less precise outputs.

System-wide signaling distortion therefore arises from a common structural shift that affects every membrane-dependent process. As packing becomes irregular and fluidity exceeds controlled limits, the conditions that enforce specificity and timing are lost. Signals initiate too easily, spread too broadly, and persist too long. The network remains active, but its outputs no longer correspond accurately to input because the structural framework that governs interaction and containment has been altered across the entire system.

Chapter 18

Chronic Inflammation as Failed Completion

Inflammation is not defined by activation alone. It is defined by the ability to complete a sequence that begins with disruption and ends with restoration of structure. The initiating event alters membrane integrity, releases signaling substrates, and recruits cellular responses that address the disturbance. Completion requires that these responses terminate once the structural issue is resolved and that the membrane returns to a state capable of maintaining controlled separation. Chronic inflammation emerges when this sequence initiates correctly but fails to terminate, leaving the system in a sustained state of activation that continues to draw on resources without restoring baseline conditions.

The process begins with structural disturbance at the membrane. Mechanical stress, chemical modification, or signaling overload alters lipid organization and triggers enzymatic release of fatty acids from phospholipids. These substrates are converted into signaling molecules that initiate local responses, increasing permeability, recruiting immune cells, and altering cellular behavior. This phase is necessary. It exposes the system to conditions that allow repair and containment of the initial disruption.

Completion requires a transition in substrate use and signaling output. The same membrane that provided substrates for initiation must also supply substrates that guide resolution. This involves shifting from signals that promote activation to those that reduce it, clear damaged components, and restore membrane organization. If the membrane lacks the appropriate composition to support this transition, signaling remains biased toward continued activation. The system continues to operate in a state designed for response rather than restoration.

Structural conditions determine whether this transition can occur. Membranes with sufficient organization and balanced lipid composition provide both the stability required to contain activation and the substrates needed for termination. When structure is compromised, permeability remains elevated, and signaling pathways continue to be engaged. This prevents the system from reestablishing the conditions required for completion, extending the active phase indefinitely.

Persistent activation alters cellular behavior across multiple systems. Immune cells remain engaged, producing signals that recruit additional cells and maintain the response. Endothelial membranes increase permeability, allowing continued movement of cells and molecules into affected areas. Signaling pathways remain active, altering metabolic and hormonal regulation. These changes do not resolve the initial disturbance. They sustain the response in the absence of completion.

Energy demand increases under these conditions. Maintaining an active response requires continuous production of signaling molecules, transport of substrates, and repair of ongoing damage. At the same time, structural instability increases leakage and inefficiency, requiring additional energy to maintain gradients and basic cellular functions. The system operates under sustained load, reducing its capacity to complete the processes required for resolution.

Remodeling cycles are also affected. Persistent activation increases the rate of lipid turnover, but if the available substrates do not support stable reconstruction, the membrane remains in a state of altered composition. This prevents restoration of the structural conditions required for termination, reinforcing the cycle of continued activation.

Chronic inflammation therefore represents a failure of completion rather than an excess of initiation. The system begins the response correctly but cannot transition to termination because the structural and compositional conditions required for that transition are not present. Activation persists, resources are consumed, and the membrane remains in a state that continues to generate signals rather than resolve them, because the architecture required to close the loop has not been restored.

Persistent Signaling Loops

Persistent signaling loops form when activation no longer depends on an external input and instead sustains itself through internal structural conditions. The membrane is the surface where this shift occurs. When lipid organization becomes irregular and permeability increases, signaling components encounter one another more frequently and remain associated longer than intended. What begins as a response to a discrete trigger transitions into a self-maintaining cycle, where the output of the system feeds back into its own activation pathways.

The loop begins with incomplete termination. Signaling molecules are generated and propagate through receptors and downstream pathways, but the mechanisms that normally reduce their concentration and separate interacting components do not complete their function. Lipid-derived mediators continue to be produced because the substrates remain available and the structural conditions that would shift production toward resolution are not established. Receptors remain in proximity, channels continue to cycle, and the membrane does not return to a baseline state that would reduce interaction frequency.

Structural permeability reinforces this process. Increased ion leakage alters electrical gradients, which changes the behavior of ion channels and transporters. These changes influence intracellular conditions, maintaining a state that favors continued activation. The membrane no longer isolates the internal environment from external variation. Instead, it allows fluctuations that sustain signaling activity even in the absence of new stimuli.

Reactive byproducts contribute to loop persistence. Oxidative modification of lipids generates molecules that act as additional signals, recruiting further activity and altering cellular behavior. These signals originate from the same structural instability that prevents termination, creating a feedback relationship where damage and signaling amplify one another. The membrane becomes both the source and the amplifier of the loop.

Immune involvement extends the cycle across systems. Persistent signals recruit immune cells that release additional mediators, increasing local activity and altering surrounding tissue behavior. These inputs do not resolve the original disturbance. They add new layers of signaling that maintain the loop. The boundary between local and systemic response begins to blur as signals propagate beyond their initial location.

Energy demand increases as the loop continues. Maintaining gradients, producing signaling molecules, and attempting repair all require ATP. As structural instability increases leakage and inefficiency, more energy is required to sustain basic conditions. This reduces the system's capacity to complete termination processes, further reinforcing persistence.

Remodeling cycles fail to break the loop when input composition remains unchanged. As lipids are replaced, the same structural conditions are reintroduced, preventing restoration of a stable baseline. The membrane continues to support conditions that favor interaction and signaling rather than separation and termination.

Persistent signaling loops therefore arise when structural conditions prevent the system from exiting an activated state. Increased mobility, permeability, and reactive byproducts maintain interactions that should be transient. The loop sustains itself through feedback between structure and signaling, extending activation beyond its functional purpose because the membrane no longer enforces the boundaries required to return the system to baseline.

Inadequate Resolution Substrate Availability

Resolution requires specific substrates embedded within the membrane that can be released and converted into mediators that terminate active responses. These substrates must already exist within the phospholipid structure at the moment activation occurs. If they are absent or present in insufficient proportion, the system cannot generate the signals required to shift from activation to termination. The membrane initiates the response using available components, but it lacks the material needed to complete it.

This imbalance begins with composition. Membranes enriched in substrates that favor initiation will generate signals that recruit, amplify, and sustain activity. If the proportion of omega-3–derived substrates is low, the pathways that produce resolving mediators are under-supplied. Enzymatic systems that would normally convert these substrates into termination signals remain active but underutilized, because the required inputs are not present in sufficient quantity. The system continues to produce initiation signals from dominant substrates, reinforcing the active state.

Availability is not determined at the moment of signaling. It is set during prior remodeling cycles that establish membrane composition. Each cycle determines which fatty acids are embedded within phospholipids and therefore accessible for release. When these cycles do not incorporate sufficient resolution-supporting substrates, the membrane enters activation phases without the capacity to generate corresponding termination signals. This creates a structural bias toward persistence.

Spatial distribution further limits availability. Even when resolution substrates are present, they must be located within the regions where signaling occurs. If they are unevenly distributed, localized areas of activation may lack access to the necessary components, preventing resolution in those regions. This creates heterogeneity within the membrane, where some areas complete responses while others remain active.

Competition between substrates intensifies this limitation. Enzymatic pathways that process fatty acids can act on multiple substrates, but they do not produce the same outputs from each. When initiation-favoring substrates dominate, they occupy enzymatic capacity, reducing the conversion of resolution-supporting substrates even if they are present. The balance of inputs determines which pathways are favored, and this balance is set by membrane composition rather than immediate demand.

Turnover and replenishment influence long-term capacity. Resolution substrates that are used during signaling must be replaced through remodeling cycles to maintain availability for future events. If replenishment is insufficient, each cycle of activation reduces the system's ability to complete subsequent responses. Over time, this leads to a progressive decline in resolution capacity.

Energy availability constrains these processes. Synthesis, incorporation, and enzymatic conversion all require ATP. When energy supply is limited, the system prioritizes immediate survival functions, reducing the resources available for maintaining substrate balance. This further limits the ability to generate resolution signals when needed.

Inadequate resolution substrate availability therefore reflects a structural limitation embedded within the membrane. The system can initiate responses but cannot complete them because the components required for termination are not present in sufficient quantity or appropriate location. This imbalance sustains activation, increases resource demand, and prevents restoration of baseline conditions because the membrane lacks the materials needed to close the signaling sequence it has begun.

Immune System Misalignment

Immune function depends on the ability to distinguish between what should be engaged and what should be ignored, then to terminate that engagement once the task is complete. This discrimination is executed at membrane interfaces where receptors detect signals, assemble into complexes, and initiate downstream responses. When membrane structure drifts away from controlled organization, the conditions that govern recognition, activation, and termination shift. The immune system does not lose its components. It loses alignment between input and response.

Recognition is the first point of failure. Immune receptors rely on spatial organization within the membrane to interpret signals correctly. Clustering must occur within defined domains to confirm that a stimulus is sufficient to warrant activation. When membrane fluidity increases beyond controlled limits, receptors encounter one another more frequently and outside of structured regions. This lowers activation thresholds and increases the likelihood of engagement in response to weak or ambiguous signals. At the same time, irregular packing alters how ligands interact with receptors, reducing the precision of detection. The system begins to respond to inputs that would normally be filtered out.

Activation follows this altered recognition. Once engaged, signaling pathways amplify the response through coordinated interactions between membrane-bound and intracellular components. Structural inconsistency affects how these interactions propagate. Some regions amplify signals excessively due to increased mobility, while others fail to sustain them due to lack of stable clustering. The result is uneven activation, where the magnitude and distribution of the response no longer reflect the original stimulus.

Termination is impaired under these conditions. Resolution requires separation of signaling complexes and the generation of mediators that reduce activity and restore baseline conditions. When membrane structure does not support controlled disassembly, signaling components remain associated longer than intended. At the same time, inadequate availability of resolution substrates limits the production of signals that would normally guide termination. The response persists even after the initial trigger is no longer present.

Boundary function becomes less distinct. Immune cells depend on membrane integrity to maintain separation between internal and external environments, as well as between self and non-self. Increased permeability and structural irregularity blur these boundaries, allowing signals and molecules to cross in ways that alter how cells interpret their surroundings. This can lead to engagement with targets that should remain ignored or failure to respond appropriately to actual threats.

Communication between immune cells is also affected. Cytokine signaling and cell-to-cell interactions rely on consistent membrane behavior to transmit information accurately. When structure varies, the same signal can produce different responses depending on local conditions. This reduces coordination across the immune network, leading to responses that are either exaggerated or insufficient.

Energy demand increases as the system attempts to maintain activity under unstable conditions. Persistent signaling, increased transport activity, and ongoing repair processes require continuous ATP input. This diverts resources from resolution and restoration, reinforcing the state of misalignment.

Remodeling cycles influence whether alignment can be restored. If membrane composition shifts toward a structure that supports controlled packing and balanced fluidity, receptor behavior and signaling dynamics return to a more precise state. If destabilizing inputs persist, remodeling reinforces the same conditions that drive misalignment, preventing correction.

Immune system misalignment therefore arises from structural conditions that alter how signals are detected, processed, and terminated. The system remains active, but its responses no longer correspond accurately to input because the membrane environment that governs interaction and interpretation has lost the consistency required for precise discrimination and controlled completion.

Tissue-Level Consequences

When membrane structure shifts across a population of cells, the effects no longer remain confined to individual signaling events. They scale into tissue behavior because every cell within that environment operates under the same altered constraints. The membrane defines permeability, signaling precision, and energy efficiency at the cellular level. When these properties drift, the coordination between cells begins to degrade, and the tissue loses its ability to maintain stable function under load.

Barrier tissues are affected first because they depend directly on controlled permeability. Epithelial and endothelial layers rely on tightly regulated membranes to maintain separation between compartments. When packing density decreases and permeability increases, ions, water, and signaling molecules cross more freely. This alters pressure gradients and fluid balance, leading to leakage and swelling within the tissue. Junctional integrity becomes harder to maintain because the underlying membrane no longer supports consistent alignment. The barrier becomes inconsistent rather than uniformly compromised, with regions of higher and lower permeability that disrupt overall function.

Signal coordination between cells becomes less reliable. In a stable system, signals propagate in a controlled manner, allowing groups of cells to respond together. When membrane properties vary, identical signals produce different responses depending on local conditions. Some cells activate rapidly, others respond weakly, and some remain active longer than intended. This desynchronization disrupts tissue-level processes that depend on timing, such as coordinated contraction, secretion, or immune response. The tissue begins to operate with internal variability rather than unified output.

Energy demand increases across the tissue as each cell compensates for increased leakage and signaling noise. Maintaining ion gradients requires more active transport, and persistent signaling loops consume additional resources. Cells allocate more energy toward maintaining basic conditions and less toward specialized functions. Over time, this reduces the overall efficiency of the tissue, limiting its ability to perform its primary role.

Structural integrity declines under mechanical stress. Tissues experience continuous forces from movement, pressure, and flow. When individual cell membranes cannot distribute these forces effectively, stress concentrates at points of weakness. This leads to micro-level disruptions that accumulate, altering tissue architecture. Cells may detach, deform, or fail to maintain proper orientation, affecting how the tissue responds to load and how signals are transmitted across it.

Inflammatory signaling becomes embedded within the tissue environment. Persistent activation at the cellular level leads to continuous release of mediators that affect neighboring cells. This creates a local environment where signaling remains elevated even in the absence of an external trigger. The tissue shifts toward a state where baseline conditions include ongoing activation, altering how it responds to new inputs.

Repair processes become less effective. Tissue maintenance depends on the ability to remove damaged components and replace them with functional ones. When membrane instability persists, newly formed cells inherit the same structural conditions, preventing full restoration.

Remodeling cycles operate, but they reproduce the existing state rather than correcting it, embedding instability into the tissue over time.

Communication with other systems becomes distorted. Hormonal, neural, and immune signals entering the tissue are interpreted through membranes that no longer provide consistent conditions. This alters how external inputs are translated into cellular responses, affecting integration with broader physiological systems. The tissue no longer responds predictably to systemic regulation.

Tissue-level consequences therefore reflect the aggregation of cellular instability into a larger system. Variability in permeability, signaling, and energy use spreads across the cellular population, disrupting coordination and reducing functional capacity. The tissue remains active, but its behavior becomes less precise and more energetically costly because the structural conditions that allow cells to operate as a coordinated unit are no longer maintained.

Chapter 19

Metabolic Disease as Structural Failure

Metabolic disease does not begin as an isolated failure of glucose handling, hormone signaling, or energy production. It emerges from a shift in membrane structure that alters how substrates are transported, how receptors respond, and how gradients are maintained. The membrane defines the conditions under which metabolism operates. When those conditions become inconsistent, metabolic pathways no longer produce outputs that match input. The system continues to process substrates, but it does so within an environment that distorts timing, sensitivity, and efficiency.

Fuel handling is the first layer affected. Transport of glucose, fatty acids, and amino acids depends on membrane proteins that require a stable lipid environment to function correctly. When packing density decreases and permeability increases, gradients that drive transport weaken, and the behavior of transporters becomes less predictable. Substrates either fail to enter cells at the required rate or enter without proper regulation. This disrupts the balance between availability and utilization, leading to accumulation in circulation and inconsistent uptake across tissues.

Hormonal signaling reflects these structural changes. Receptors embedded within the membrane rely on controlled fluidity and organized domains to initiate and propagate signals. When the membrane becomes either too rigid or too fluid, receptor behavior shifts. In the case of insulin signaling, altered membrane composition affects how receptors cluster and how downstream pathways are activated. The result is a reduced ability to translate circulating signals into cellular responses. Hormones remain present, but their effect is diminished because the structural environment required for signal transmission is no longer intact.

Mitochondrial function is directly influenced by membrane integrity. The inner mitochondrial membrane must maintain tight control over proton gradients to produce ATP efficiently. Increased permeability and altered lipid composition allow protons to leak, reducing the efficiency of energy conversion. This forces the system to increase substrate oxidation to maintain output, raising metabolic demand while producing less usable energy. Over time, this inefficiency contributes to fatigue at the cellular level and reduces the capacity for adaptive responses.

Energy distribution across the system becomes uneven. Some tissues compensate by increasing uptake and utilization, while others remain resistant due to impaired transport and signaling. This creates a state where substrates accumulate in circulation while certain cells operate under relative scarcity. The imbalance is not due to lack of input but to inconsistent structural conditions that determine how that input is processed.

Inflammatory signaling integrates with these changes. Persistent membrane instability promotes ongoing activation of signaling pathways that alter metabolic regulation. These signals interfere with normal hormonal responses and further disrupt substrate handling. The system enters a state where metabolic and inflammatory processes reinforce one another, each amplifying the effects of the other.

Remodeling cycles continue to operate within this altered state. If the input pool of lipids does not support stable reconstruction, each cycle reinforces the same structural conditions that produced the dysfunction. The membrane does not return to a configuration that supports efficient metabolism. Instead, it stabilizes at a new baseline where inefficiency is embedded into the system.

Energy demand increases as compensation mechanisms attempt to maintain function. Greater effort is required to sustain gradients, process substrates, and manage signaling noise. This reduces overall efficiency and limits the system's ability to respond to additional stress. The gap between input and usable output widens, even as total substrate availability remains high.

Metabolic disease therefore reflects a structural failure at the level of the membrane. The processes responsible for handling fuel, transmitting signals, and producing energy continue to operate, but they do so within an environment that no longer supports precision or efficiency. As a result, the system produces outputs that do not align with input because the architecture that governs metabolic behavior has shifted away from the conditions required for controlled and coordinated function.

Insulin Resistance as Receptor Environment Failure

Insulin resistance emerges when the membrane environment no longer supports the sequence of events required for receptor activation and signal transmission. The insulin receptor does not operate as an isolated switch. It depends on spatial organization within the bilayer, lateral mobility to assemble signaling complexes, and a stable lipid context that maintains its conformation. When membrane composition drifts, these conditions change, and the receptor remains present but no longer produces the expected output in response to insulin binding.

Activation begins with receptor clustering. Insulin binding increases the likelihood that receptors come into proximity and transition into an active state. This process requires controlled fluidity. If the membrane becomes too rigid, receptors cannot move into position efficiently, and activation is reduced. If too fluid, receptors encounter one another too frequently and outside of organized domains, producing unstable or incomplete activation. In both cases, the signal that initiates downstream pathways becomes inconsistent, reducing the effectiveness of the response.

The surrounding lipid environment determines how the receptor changes shape during activation. Conformational transitions depend on a membrane that provides both support and flexibility. Altered packing density changes how forces are distributed across the receptor, affecting its ability to shift between inactive and active states. This leads to a reduction in signaling precision, where the receptor binds insulin but fails to propagate the signal with sufficient strength or duration.

Signal propagation requires the recruitment of downstream proteins to the membrane. These interactions occur within defined regions where lipid composition supports the assembly of signaling complexes. When membrane organization is disrupted, these regions become unstable. Proteins fail to localize correctly, and the sequence of interactions required for signal transmission is interrupted. The pathway does not fail completely. It becomes inefficient, requiring higher levels of insulin to achieve the same effect.

Permeability and electrical stability influence intracellular conditions that modulate signaling. Increased leakage alters ion gradients and cellular energy status, affecting kinase activity and phosphorylation events that are central to insulin signaling. These changes reduce the responsiveness of the pathway, further contributing to resistance.

Chronic signaling distortion compounds the problem. Persistent activation of other pathways, driven by structural instability, interferes with insulin signaling by altering the availability and activity of shared components. This creates competition within the signaling network, reducing the ability of insulin to produce a clear and dominant response.

Energy availability plays a limiting role. Signal transduction requires ATP for phosphorylation and transport processes. When mitochondrial efficiency declines due to membrane instability, the energy required to sustain signaling becomes constrained. This reduces the capacity of the cell to respond even when receptors are activated.

Remodeling cycles determine whether this condition persists. If membrane composition continues to reflect inputs that disrupt packing and organization, the receptor environment remains suboptimal. Replacement of lipids with those that support stable structure gradually restores the conditions required for proper signaling, but this process depends on sustained input and active turnover.

Insulin resistance therefore reflects a failure of the receptor environment rather than the absence of receptors or hormone. The signal is present, and the receptor can bind it, but the structural conditions required to convert that binding into a coordinated intracellular response are not maintained. The system compensates by increasing insulin levels, but the underlying issue remains because the membrane no longer provides the framework necessary for precise and efficient signal transmission.

Obesity as Lipid Mismanagement, Not Excess

Obesity reflects a breakdown in how lipids are handled, directed, and incorporated into structure rather than a simple accumulation of surplus energy. The body is designed to store lipids as part of a controlled system where intake, transport, storage, and mobilization remain coordinated. Adipose tissue functions as a regulated buffer, absorbing fluctuations in substrate availability and releasing stored fuel when required. This system depends on membrane integrity across multiple tissues, because transporters, receptors, and enzymes that govern lipid flow all operate within lipid environments. When those environments become unstable, the routing of lipids shifts, and storage expands as a consequence of misallocation rather than uncontrolled intake.

Lipid entry into adipose tissue is not passive. It depends on signals that direct fatty acids toward storage or oxidation. When membrane composition alters receptor behavior, these signals become distorted. Insulin signaling, which normally coordinates uptake and storage, becomes inconsistent, leading to a state where adipose tissue continues to receive lipids while other tissues fail to access them efficiently. Circulating substrates remain elevated, and adipose tissue expands because it is one of the few compartments still capable of absorbing excess input under these conditions.

Adipocyte structure changes as storage increases. The membrane must expand to accommodate larger lipid droplets, and its composition determines whether this expansion can occur without loss of function. When structural stability is compromised, the cell experiences mechanical stress and increased permeability. This alters signaling within the adipocyte and promotes the release of inflammatory mediators that affect neighboring cells and surrounding tissue. The expansion of adipose tissue therefore includes a shift in its signaling behavior, not just its size.

Lipid mobilization becomes impaired under these conditions. Releasing stored fatty acids requires coordinated signaling and intact membrane function. When receptor responsiveness declines and intracellular signaling becomes inconsistent, the ability to access stored energy decreases. This creates a state where lipids are both accumulated and unavailable, forcing reliance on other substrates while storage continues to grow.

Ectopic deposition emerges as a secondary effect. When adipose tissue reaches its functional limits or loses the ability to expand in a controlled manner, lipids are redirected into other tissues such as liver and muscle. These tissues are not structured for long-term storage, and the presence of excess lipid alters their membrane composition and function. This further disrupts signaling and energy production, reinforcing the underlying problem.

Energy balance appears distorted because intake and storage no longer correspond to utilization. The system continues to take in and process substrates, but distribution is uneven. Some compartments accumulate excess, while others operate under restricted access. This mismatch creates the appearance of surplus alongside functional deficiency.

Inflammatory signaling integrates with lipid mismanagement. As adipose tissue expands and membrane integrity declines, local signaling shifts toward a persistent activated state. These signals influence systemic metabolism, altering how other tissues respond to substrates and hormones. The result is a feedback loop where structural instability promotes further misallocation of lipids.

Remodeling cycles determine the direction of change. If membrane composition remains dominated by inputs that reduce stability, each cycle reinforces the conditions that drive mismanagement. If inputs shift toward lipids that support controlled packing and signaling, the system gradually restores coordination between storage and utilization. Adipose tissue then returns to its role as a regulated buffer rather than a continuously expanding compartment.

Obesity therefore represents a failure in the organization and control of lipid flow. Storage increases because the system can no longer direct lipids with precision, not because the body is incapable of regulating intake alone. The expansion of adipose tissue reflects an attempt to contain misallocated substrates within a structure designed for storage, while the underlying issue remains rooted in the membrane environments that govern how lipids are processed, distributed, and accessed across the system.

Mitochondrial Inefficiency and Energy Leakage

Mitochondrial output depends on the ability to confine and control a proton gradient across the inner membrane. Electron transport moves charge through a series of complexes, and that movement is used to pump protons into the intermembrane space. The separation of charge creates a gradient that stores potential energy. ATP synthesis draws on that gradient by allowing protons to flow back through a controlled channel. The entire process is defined by containment. When the membrane holds the gradient tightly, energy is captured and converted with high efficiency. When containment weakens, protons return without passing through ATP synthase, and the stored energy dissipates as heat rather than being converted into usable work.

Membrane composition determines how well this gradient is maintained. The inner mitochondrial membrane requires tight packing and low permeability to prevent uncontrolled proton movement. Cardiolipin plays a central role by stabilizing the structure of the electron transport complexes and maintaining the organization of the membrane. When lipid composition shifts away from this configuration, the membrane becomes more permissive. Small increases in permeability are enough to allow protons to bypass ATP synthase, reducing the amount of energy captured per unit of substrate oxidized.

Electron transport becomes less stable under these conditions. The complexes rely on precise spatial relationships to transfer electrons efficiently. When the membrane environment changes, these relationships are disrupted, and electron flow becomes less consistent. This increases the likelihood that electrons escape the chain prematurely, interacting with oxygen to form reactive species. These reactions do not contribute to ATP production but instead create additional stress that the system must manage.

The system compensates by increasing throughput. To maintain ATP levels, more substrate must be oxidized to offset the loss of efficiency. This raises oxygen consumption and increases the load on the electron transport chain, further elevating the chance of electron leakage. The cycle reinforces itself. Reduced efficiency leads to higher demand, which increases instability and further reduces efficiency.

Heat production increases as a direct result of proton leakage. Energy that would normally be captured in ATP is released during uncontrolled proton flow. While some degree of uncoupling is used intentionally in specific tissues, widespread leakage represents a loss of control rather than a regulated process. The system expends resources without generating proportional output.

Cellular energy balance shifts under these conditions. ATP availability becomes less stable, affecting processes that depend on consistent energy supply. Transport systems, biosynthetic pathways, and signaling mechanisms all require ATP to function correctly. Variability in energy production leads to variability in these processes, contributing to broader system instability.

Mitochondrial dynamics are affected as well. Fusion and fission processes depend on membrane integrity and energy availability. When the membrane environment is compromised, these processes become less effective at maintaining functional mitochondria. Damaged components persist longer, and the overall quality of the mitochondrial population declines.

Repair and turnover systems are placed under increased demand. Reactive species generated from electron leakage damage lipids, proteins, and mitochondrial DNA. The system must allocate resources to repair or remove these components, further diverting energy away from productive work. If repair cannot keep pace with damage, dysfunction accumulates.

Mitochondrial inefficiency therefore reflects a failure to maintain the structural conditions required for gradient containment and controlled energy conversion. The machinery remains present and active, but the membrane no longer provides the isolation needed to preserve potential energy. As a result, substrate oxidation increases while usable output declines, and energy is lost through pathways that bypass the mechanisms designed to capture it.

System-Wide Instability

Once membrane structure drifts across multiple tissues, instability no longer appears as isolated dysfunction. It becomes a system-level condition where inputs are processed differently depending on local membrane state, producing outputs that no longer align across organs. The body relies on coordinated signaling, consistent transport, and predictable energy distribution. When these underlying conditions vary, the system loses synchronization. Each tissue continues to operate, but it does so under slightly different rules, and the integration that normally holds physiology together begins to fragment.

Signal interpretation becomes inconsistent. Hormones and circulating mediators arrive with a defined concentration and timing, but their effects depend on how receptors respond within each tissue. When membrane composition differs, receptor behavior shifts. One tissue may respond strongly, another weakly, and a third may remain active longer than intended. The signal itself has not changed, but the response profile becomes uneven. This creates conflicting outputs, where the same input drives opposing actions in different parts of the system.

Transport loses coherence. Movement of substrates, ions, and signaling molecules depends on gradients and membrane permeability. When these properties vary, distribution becomes irregular. Some tissues accumulate substrates while others remain under-supplied despite adequate circulation. The imbalance is not due to supply limitations but to differences in how membranes allow or restrict movement. This distorts nutrient availability at the cellular level and disrupts the alignment between intake and utilization.

Energy allocation becomes unstable. Mitochondrial inefficiency in one tissue increases demand for substrates, while resistance to uptake in another limits its ability to use available fuel. The system attempts to compensate by adjusting hormonal output and substrate release, but these adjustments are interpreted differently across tissues. The result is a state where energy is present but not evenly accessible, leading to simultaneous accumulation and deficit within different compartments.

Feedback loops amplify instability. Persistent signaling from one tissue influences the behavior of others, but when responses are inconsistent, these signals do not produce corrective effects. Instead, they reinforce existing imbalances. A signal intended to reduce activity in one area may fail to suppress it while altering function elsewhere, creating cycles that maintain or increase system-wide disruption.

Temporal coordination breaks down. Many processes depend on timing, including hormone release, metabolic transitions, and repair cycles. When membrane-dependent signaling varies, the onset and duration of responses shift. Processes that should occur in sequence begin to overlap or occur out of order, reducing efficiency and increasing the likelihood of interference between pathways.

Structural variability becomes self-reinforcing. Remodeling cycles operate continuously, incorporating available lipids into membranes. If the input environment does not support stable composition, each cycle reproduces the same conditions that generated instability. Over time, variability becomes embedded into the system, making spontaneous correction unlikely without a shift in structural inputs.

Communication between systems loses precision. Neural, endocrine, and immune pathways depend on consistent signal transmission and interpretation. When membrane properties differ across tissues, these systems cannot coordinate effectively. Signals are still transmitted, but their meaning changes as they pass through different environments, reducing the reliability of system-wide regulation.

System-wide instability therefore reflects the loss of a shared structural baseline across tissues. The body no longer operates as a unified system with coordinated responses to input. Instead, it becomes a collection of compartments responding independently, each shaped by its local membrane conditions. The processes that maintain balance remain active, but without consistent structural constraints, their outputs diverge, and the system loses the coherence required for stable function.

PART VI

REBUILDING LIPID ARCHITECTURE

Chapter 20

Removing Structural Interference

Restoring function begins by removing inputs that disrupt membrane organization rather than by forcing output through stimulation or compensation. Every membrane is built from available lipids, and those lipids determine packing density, permeability, and signaling behavior. When the input pool is dominated by structures that introduce instability, each remodeling cycle reinforces the same conditions that produced dysfunction. Removing structural interference shifts the substrate pool, allowing subsequent turnover to rebuild membranes with properties that support controlled transport, receptor function, and energy containment. The process is not immediate because existing membranes persist until they are replaced, but the direction of change is set by what is no longer being incorporated.

Industrial lipid exposure represents a primary source of interference. Highly unsaturated fatty acids with multiple double bonds increase susceptibility to oxidation and reduce packing stability when incorporated into membranes. As these lipids accumulate, they alter fluidity and increase variability across tissues. Oxidized derivatives further disrupt signaling by introducing reactive species into the membrane environment. Removing these inputs reduces the rate at which unstable structures are introduced, lowering both direct structural disruption and secondary oxidative stress.

Repeated thermal and chemical modification of fats compounds this effect. Heating alters lipid structure, producing compounds that do not integrate into membranes in a controlled manner. These altered lipids increase permeability and interfere with normal signaling processes once incorporated. Eliminating sources of repeatedly heated or chemically modified fats reduces the burden of these structurally inconsistent inputs, allowing the membrane to maintain more uniform properties across tissues.

Excessive intake of highly unsaturated substrates without sufficient structural context introduces another layer of interference. Polyunsaturated fatty acids are required for specific signaling roles, but their integration into membranes must remain balanced with lipids that provide stability. When this balance shifts, membranes become more permissive and less capable of maintaining gradients and organized signaling domains. Adjusting intake toward a composition that supports both function and stability reduces variability in membrane behavior.

Oxidative load interacts directly with membrane composition. Reactive species target double bonds within lipids, initiating chain reactions that damage surrounding structures. As damage accumulates, membrane integrity declines, and signaling becomes less precise. Reducing sources of oxidative stress and limiting exposure to conditions that accelerate lipid oxidation decreases the rate of structural degradation, allowing repair and remodeling processes to operate more effectively.

Nutrient availability influences how well membranes can be maintained and repaired. Components required for lipid synthesis, antioxidant defense, and energy production must be present in sufficient quantities to support turnover. Without these inputs, even the removal of interfering lipids cannot fully restore structure because the system lacks the materials and energy required for reconstruction. Ensuring adequate supply supports the transition from removal to rebuilding.

Remodeling cycles govern the pace of change. Cells continuously replace membrane components through processes that integrate new lipids and remove damaged ones. The rate of turnover varies by tissue, meaning that structural improvement occurs gradually and unevenly across the system. Tissues with higher turnover respond more quickly, while others require sustained input over longer periods to reflect changes in composition.

Signal clarity improves as structural interference is reduced. Receptors operate within more consistent environments, allowing activation and termination to align more closely with input. Transport systems regain the ability to maintain gradients, and mitochondrial membranes recover the capacity to contain energy. These changes do not occur in isolation.

They propagate across tissues as remodeling progresses, restoring coordination between systems.

Removing structural interference therefore establishes the conditions required for recovery without directly forcing specific outcomes. By altering the composition of inputs, the system is allowed to rebuild according to its inherent design. Membranes regain the properties needed to support controlled exchange, precise signaling, and efficient energy use, and the processes that depend on these properties begin to realign as structural consistency is restored.

Eliminating Unstable Lipid Inputs

Membrane structure reflects the lipid pool available at the time of remodeling. Every cycle of turnover draws from circulating substrates and incorporates them into the bilayer, where their physical properties determine packing, permeability, and signaling behavior. When the input pool contains lipids that disrupt stable organization, each cycle embeds those properties into the membrane. Eliminating unstable lipid inputs changes the composition of that pool, reducing the probability that new membranes will be built with characteristics that increase variability and leakage.

Highly unsaturated fatty acids introduce structural irregularity when present in excess. Multiple double bonds create kinks that prevent tight packing, increasing spacing between adjacent lipids and raising baseline permeability. This alters how ions and small molecules move across the membrane and changes the environment in which receptors and transporters operate. While these lipids serve specific signaling roles, their overrepresentation shifts the balance away from structural containment. Reducing their intake lowers their incorporation rate, allowing membranes to rebuild with a higher proportion of lipids that support consistent packing.

Oxidized lipids represent a direct form of structural interference. Exposure to heat, light, or reactive species modifies fatty acids, producing compounds that integrate poorly into membranes. Once incorporated, these altered lipids disrupt local organization and increase the likelihood of further reactions within the bilayer. They also interfere with protein function by altering the surrounding lipid environment. Eliminating sources of oxidized fats reduces the introduction of these disruptive elements, limiting both immediate structural effects and downstream propagation of damage.

Repeated heating amplifies lipid instability. Thermal processing alters the chemical structure of fats, generating byproducts that differ from their original form. These compounds do not behave predictably when integrated into membranes, contributing to variability in fluidity and signaling. Avoiding fats that have undergone repeated heating reduces the presence of these altered structures in the input pool.

The balance between lipid classes determines overall membrane behavior. Saturated and monounsaturated fats provide structural stability and controlled flexibility, while polyunsaturated fats contribute to signaling capacity. When intake skews heavily toward highly unsaturated lipids, membranes become more permissive and less consistent across tissues. Adjusting this balance shifts the baseline properties of newly formed membranes, restoring a combination of stability and function that supports controlled exchange and signaling precision.

Circulating lipids influence remodeling continuously. Lipoprotein transport systems deliver fatty acids to tissues, where they are either oxidized or incorporated into membranes. The composition of these carriers reflects dietary input and endogenous processing. By altering the types of lipids entering circulation, the distribution of substrates available for membrane construction changes, affecting all tissues over time.

Turnover rates determine how quickly elimination of unstable inputs produces observable changes. Tissues with rapid membrane replacement adjust more quickly, while those with slower turnover require sustained periods of altered input to reflect new composition. This creates a staggered pattern of improvement, where some functions stabilize earlier than others.

Signal behavior improves as unstable inputs are removed. Receptor activity becomes more consistent because the surrounding lipid environment supports proper clustering and conformational change. Transport systems regain the ability to maintain gradients with less energy expenditure. Mitochondrial membranes reduce leakage, improving energy capture efficiency. These effects arise from changes in structure rather than direct manipulation of signaling pathways.

Eliminating unstable lipid inputs therefore shifts the foundational conditions under which cellular processes operate. By reducing the incorporation of lipids that disrupt packing and increase variability, the system rebuilds membranes that support containment, precise signaling, and efficient energy use. The outcome reflects the gradual replacement of unstable structures with configurations that restore consistency across tissues.

Reducing Oxidative Load on Membranes

Membrane stability depends not only on the types of lipids incorporated but on the rate at which those lipids are chemically altered after incorporation. Oxidation targets the weakest points in the structure, which are the double bonds within unsaturated fatty acids. When reactive species interact with these sites, they initiate chain reactions that propagate across the bilayer, modifying adjacent lipids and altering the physical properties of the membrane. As this process continues, packing becomes less uniform, permeability increases, and the behavior of embedded proteins shifts. Reducing oxidative load lowers the frequency of these reactions, allowing membranes to maintain their structural integrity over time.

The initiation of lipid oxidation occurs when reactive species encounter susceptible lipids. These species arise from normal metabolic activity, particularly within mitochondria, but their production increases when electron transport becomes unstable or when external stressors add to the burden. Once initiated, lipid peroxidation proceeds through a series of reactions that generate additional reactive intermediates, extending damage beyond the initial site. Interrupting this process requires limiting both the generation of reactive species and the availability of highly susceptible substrates within the membrane.

Membrane composition determines vulnerability. Lipids with multiple double bonds provide more sites for oxidative attack, increasing the likelihood that a reaction will begin and propagate. When these lipids dominate the membrane, even moderate levels of reactive species can produce widespread damage. Shifting composition toward structures that are less prone to oxidation reduces the number of initiation points, lowering the probability that chain reactions will occur.

Antioxidant systems function within the membrane to terminate these reactions. Lipid-soluble compounds positioned within the bilayer intercept reactive intermediates, preventing the spread of oxidation to neighboring lipids. The effectiveness of these systems depends on both their concentration and their distribution within the membrane. When oxidative load exceeds the capacity of these defenses, damage accumulates and alters membrane behavior.

Mitochondrial activity contributes significantly to oxidative load. Inefficient electron transport increases the leakage of electrons that react with oxygen to form reactive species. As membrane integrity declines, this leakage becomes more pronounced, creating a feedback loop where oxidative damage further impairs mitochondrial function. Improving membrane conditions reduces electron leakage, lowering the internal generation of reactive species and decreasing the overall burden on the system.

External inputs influence oxidative exposure. Light, heat, and chemically altered fats introduce oxidized compounds directly into the system, adding to the internal load. These compounds integrate into membranes and act as starting points for further reactions. Reducing exposure to these inputs decreases the number of external initiation sites, allowing endogenous systems to manage oxidative processes more effectively.

Repair and replacement processes operate continuously to remove damaged lipids and incorporate new ones. The rate at which these processes restore membrane integrity depends on the balance between damage and repair. When oxidative load is reduced, repair mechanisms can keep pace with or exceed the rate of damage, allowing membranes to return toward a more stable configuration.

Signal precision improves as oxidative load decreases. Receptors embedded within membranes operate more consistently when the surrounding lipid environment is intact. Transport systems maintain gradients with less energy expenditure, and mitochondrial membranes preserve the gradients required for efficient ATP production. These changes arise from the preservation of structure rather than direct modulation of signaling pathways.

Reducing oxidative load on membranes therefore stabilizes the physical environment that underlies cellular function. By limiting both the initiation and propagation of lipid oxidation, the system maintains uniform packing, controlled permeability, and reliable protein behavior. This allows signaling, transport, and energy production processes to operate within conditions that support precision and efficiency across tissues.

Stopping Continuous Remodeling into Weakness

Membranes are not static structures. They are continuously dismantled and rebuilt through remodeling cycles that replace existing lipids with those available in circulation. This process allows adaptation, but it also means that structural instability can become self-reinforcing. When the input pool is dominated by lipids that reduce packing density, increase susceptibility to oxidation, or disrupt domain organization, each cycle embeds those properties into newly formed membranes. The system does not fail because it stops remodeling. It fails because remodeling continues in the wrong direction.

The direction of remodeling is determined by substrate availability. Circulating fatty acids delivered through lipoproteins are incorporated into membranes based on local demand and enzymatic activity. When these substrates favor instability, the resulting membranes inherit increased permeability and reduced structural coherence. This alters receptor behavior, transport efficiency, and energy containment, which in turn influences how substrates are processed and redistributed. The system begins to feed its own instability by generating conditions that maintain the same input profile.

Enzymatic remodeling pathways operate without evaluating structural outcomes. They exchange fatty acids within phospholipids based on availability and kinetic preference rather than functional optimization. When unstable lipids are abundant, they are incorporated repeatedly, displacing more stable components. This shifts the baseline composition of membranes across tissues, embedding variability into the system. The process continues as long as the input pool remains unchanged.

Oxidative damage accelerates this cycle. Damaged lipids are removed and replaced, but if the replacement pool contains the same susceptible structures, the new membrane remains vulnerable. Each cycle removes damaged components but reintroduces the conditions that caused the damage. This creates a loop where turnover increases without improving stability, consuming energy while failing to restore function.

Stopping this progression requires altering the composition of available substrates so that each remodeling cycle produces a more stable outcome. When the input pool shifts toward lipids that support tighter packing and controlled fluidity, newly formed membranes begin to reflect these properties. Over time, repeated cycles replace unstable structures with configurations that maintain gradients, support receptor organization, and resist oxidative disruption.

Turnover rates determine how quickly this transition occurs. Tissues with rapid membrane replacement respond sooner, while those with slower turnover require sustained changes in substrate availability to achieve similar results. The process is cumulative. Each cycle contributes incrementally to the overall structure, gradually shifting the system toward stability.

Signal behavior stabilizes as remodeling direction changes. Receptors operate within more consistent environments, reducing variability in activation and termination. Transport systems regain efficiency as gradients are maintained with less leakage. Mitochondrial membranes improve containment, increasing the proportion of substrate energy captured as ATP.

Energy demand decreases as stability improves. Fewer resources are required to maintain gradients, repair damage, and compensate for signaling noise. This allows the system to allocate energy toward productive processes rather than continuous correction of instability.

Stopping continuous remodeling into weakness therefore depends on controlling the inputs that define membrane construction. By shifting the substrate pool, each cycle of turnover becomes a step toward improved structure rather than a repetition of dysfunction. The system does not need to be forced into correction. It rebuilds itself according to the materials available, and when those materials support stability, the outcomes align with efficient and coordinated function.

Creating Conditions for Stabilization

Stabilization does not begin with forcing specific outputs. It begins with restoring the baseline conditions that allow membranes to maintain consistent structure across tissues. The system organizes itself around what is physically possible within the lipid environment. When that environment supports tight packing, controlled fluidity, and resistance to degradation, transport, signaling, and energy production align without requiring constant compensation. Creating these conditions means establishing a substrate pool and internal environment where stable structures can form and persist through successive remodeling cycles.

The lipid composition of membranes must support both containment and flexibility. Saturated fatty acids provide linear structure that allows close packing and reduces baseline permeability. Monounsaturated fatty acids introduce controlled spacing that prevents excessive rigidity while maintaining coherence. Together, these lipids define a range of fluidity where receptors can move and interact without losing organization.

When this balance is established, membranes maintain gradients more effectively, and embedded proteins operate within predictable mechanical constraints.

Cholesterol contributes to this stability by regulating spacing between phospholipids. It reduces excessive fluidity when unsaturated lipids are present and prevents rigid packing when saturation is high. This allows membranes to maintain consistent properties across temperature and pressure changes. Without sufficient cholesterol, membranes become more susceptible to fluctuations in composition, leading to variability in permeability and signaling behavior.

The internal oxidative environment must be controlled to preserve these structures once formed. Even stable lipid compositions degrade under high oxidative load. Antioxidant systems positioned within the membrane interrupt chain reactions that would otherwise propagate damage. The effectiveness of these systems depends on both availability and distribution, ensuring that reactive intermediates are neutralized before they alter surrounding lipids.

Energy availability influences the ability to maintain stability. ATP is required to sustain ion gradients, drive transport systems, and support repair processes. When mitochondrial membranes contain gradients efficiently, energy production remains consistent, allowing the system to maintain structure without excessive strain. When energy is limited, maintenance processes become less effective, and instability accumulates.

Enzymatic processes that govern lipid remodeling respond to substrate availability and local conditions. When the input pool favors stable lipids, these enzymes incorporate components that reinforce membrane integrity. Over time, repeated cycles of incorporation and replacement shift the overall composition toward structures that maintain consistent behavior across tissues.

Environmental inputs must align with these structural requirements. Exposure to oxidized fats, repeated thermal processing, and other sources of chemically altered lipids introduces components that disrupt stability. Reducing these inputs lowers the burden on repair systems and prevents the introduction of structures that would counteract stabilization.

Signal clarity improves as conditions stabilize. Receptors operate within organized domains, allowing activation and termination to correspond more closely to input. Transport systems maintain gradients with reduced energy expenditure, and mitochondrial membranes preserve the conditions required for efficient ATP production. These changes occur as a result of improved structure rather than direct manipulation of signaling pathways.

Time governs the transition. Membranes are replaced incrementally, and stabilization emerges as the cumulative effect of many remodeling cycles. Tissues with higher turnover rates reflect changes sooner, while others require sustained conditions to achieve the same outcome. The process is continuous, with each cycle reinforcing the properties established by the current substrate pool.

Creating conditions for stabilization therefore involves aligning lipid inputs, oxidative environment, and energy availability so that membrane structure can be maintained without constant correction. When these conditions are present, the system shifts toward a state where transport, signaling, and energy production operate within consistent constraints, allowing coordinated function across tissues without the need for compensatory mechanisms.

Chapter 21

Reconstructing Membrane Integrity

Membrane integrity is not restored by a single input or isolated intervention. It is rebuilt through repeated cycles of lipid incorporation, structural organization, and selective removal of damaged components. The membrane exists as a continuously updated interface where composition determines behavior. Reconstruction begins when the input pool, oxidative environment, and energy availability align to support stable assembly. From that point forward, each remodeling cycle shifts the structure incrementally toward a configuration that maintains containment, supports signaling precision, and resists degradation under load.

The bilayer must re-establish uniform packing. Phospholipids arrange according to the properties of their fatty acid chains, and the distribution of these chains determines how tightly the membrane holds together. When stable lipids dominate, adjacent molecules align with minimal gaps, reducing passive permeability and allowing gradients to persist. This affects not only ion balance but also the mechanical behavior of the membrane, providing a consistent platform for embedded proteins. Reconstruction therefore involves replacing irregular arrangements with a more uniform lattice that supports controlled exchange.

Domain organization returns as composition stabilizes. Membrane microdomains form when specific lipids and proteins cluster into regions with distinct properties. These regions serve as sites for signaling, transport, and structural coordination. When lipid composition is inconsistent, these domains become unstable or fail to form altogether. As stable lipids are incorporated, the membrane regains the ability to segregate into organized regions, allowing receptors and associated proteins to localize correctly. This restores the conditions required for coordinated signal initiation and propagation.

Cholesterol distribution becomes more effective within this reconstructed environment. It positions itself between phospholipids to regulate spacing and maintain consistent fluidity. In a stable membrane, cholesterol prevents excessive movement without restricting necessary interactions. This contributes to both mechanical stability and signal fidelity, as receptors operate within an environment that supports predictable behavior.

Membrane proteins begin to function within defined constraints. Transporters, channels, and receptors depend on the surrounding lipid environment for their structure and activity. When that environment is restored, these proteins regain their ability to operate efficiently. Ion channels maintain gradients with less energy expenditure, receptors respond proportionally to stimuli, and transport systems move substrates in a controlled manner. The improvement is not due to changes in the proteins themselves but to the restoration of the conditions that allow them to function as designed.

Mitochondrial membranes follow the same principles. Reconstruction of the inner membrane improves the containment of proton gradients and stabilizes the arrangement of electron transport complexes. As leakage decreases, ATP production becomes more efficient, reducing the need for compensatory increases in substrate oxidation. This restores a more stable energy supply, which supports maintenance and repair processes throughout the cell.

Repair mechanisms operate more effectively as structural integrity improves. Damaged lipids are identified and replaced, and oxidative chain reactions are limited by a membrane that resists propagation. The rate of damage decreases, allowing repair processes to outpace degradation. Over time, this shifts the balance toward maintenance rather than continuous correction.

Intercellular consistency emerges as membranes across tissues converge toward similar structural properties. This reduces variability in signaling and transport, allowing coordinated responses to systemic inputs. Hormonal signals produce more uniform effects, and energy distribution becomes more predictable. The system begins to operate as an integrated whole rather than as a collection of independently behaving compartments.

Reconstruction proceeds through time and repetition. Each cycle of lipid turnover contributes to the overall structure, and the pace of change depends on the rate at which membranes are replaced. Sustained conditions are required to ensure that new structures are not immediately disrupted by unfavorable inputs. As stable composition becomes the default, maintenance requires less intervention, and the system holds its structure with greater efficiency.

Reconstructing membrane integrity therefore involves restoring the physical conditions that define how cells interact with their environment. By aligning composition, reducing damage, and supporting energy production, the membrane regains its role as a controlled interface. From this foundation, transport, signaling, and metabolic processes realign, producing outcomes that reflect the underlying architecture rather than compensatory adaptations to instability.

Reintroducing Stable Lipid Substrates

Membrane reconstruction depends on what is available for incorporation at the moment of remodeling. Once unstable inputs are reduced, the system requires a consistent supply of lipids that support tight packing, controlled fluidity, and resistance to degradation. These substrates do not act as signals in isolation. They become part of the membrane itself, altering its physical properties with each cycle of replacement. Reintroduction therefore defines the direction of rebuilding by determining which structures are repeatedly selected and embedded into the bilayer.

Saturated fatty acids provide the foundation for this process. Their linear structure allows adjacent lipids to align closely, reducing spacing and limiting passive permeability. As these lipids are incorporated into phospholipids, the membrane becomes more capable of maintaining ion gradients and resisting deformation under stress. This improves the baseline conditions under which transporters and receptors operate, as the surrounding environment becomes more uniform and less susceptible to fluctuation.

Monounsaturated fatty acids introduce controlled flexibility into this structure. A single double bond creates a predictable bend that prevents excessive rigidity while preserving overall packing integrity. This allows membranes to maintain mobility where it is required for receptor interaction and domain formation without losing containment. The balance between saturated and monounsaturated lipids defines a range of fluidity where both stability and function are preserved.

Cholesterol integrates with these lipids to regulate spacing and mechanical behavior. It inserts between phospholipids and adjusts local packing based on surrounding composition, preventing extremes in fluidity. As stable lipid substrates become more prevalent, cholesterol can perform this regulatory role more effectively, contributing to consistent membrane properties across different tissues and conditions.

Phospholipid synthesis reflects the availability of these substrates. Enzymatic pathways assemble phospholipids using fatty acids drawn from the circulating pool. When stable substrates dominate, newly formed phospholipids inherit properties that support membrane integrity. Over successive remodeling cycles, this shifts the overall composition toward structures that maintain gradients and support organized signaling.

Incorporation occurs gradually. Existing membranes are not replaced immediately but are remodeled through continuous turnover. Each cycle introduces a portion of new lipids while removing older or damaged components. The rate of change depends on tissue-specific turnover, meaning that some systems reflect the new substrate profile sooner than others. Sustained availability of stable lipids ensures that each cycle contributes to a consistent direction of change.

Signal behavior begins to align with these structural changes. Receptors operate within environments that allow proper clustering and conformational shifts, improving the translation of external signals into intracellular responses. Transport systems maintain gradients with reduced energy expenditure, and mitochondrial membranes contain proton gradients more effectively, increasing ATP production efficiency.

Resistance to oxidative damage increases as stable substrates replace more susceptible lipids. With fewer sites for reactive species to initiate chain reactions, the rate of membrane degradation decreases. This allows repair mechanisms to maintain integrity without being overwhelmed, reinforcing the stability established through composition.

Distribution of these substrates across tissues is mediated by lipoprotein transport systems. As circulating lipid composition changes, delivery to different organs reflects this new profile. Over time, this leads to a convergence of membrane properties across tissues, reducing variability in function and improving coordination between systems.

Reintroducing stable lipid substrates therefore provides the material basis for reconstruction. By supplying lipids that support consistent packing and controlled flexibility, the system rebuilds membranes that maintain containment, enable precise signaling, and sustain efficient energy production. The outcome emerges from repeated incorporation rather than immediate effect, as each cycle of remodeling integrates these substrates into the architecture that governs cellular behavior.

Saturated and Monounsaturated Rebuilding

Reconstruction of membrane integrity depends on re-establishing a lipid environment that can maintain both containment and controlled interaction. Saturated and monounsaturated fatty acids form the structural base that allows this to occur. Their integration into phospholipids determines how tightly the bilayer holds together, how much lateral movement is permitted, and how consistently proteins embedded within the membrane can operate. The rebuilding process is not about increasing one class in isolation. It is about restoring a ratio that produces predictable mechanical behavior across the membrane surface.

Saturated fatty acids provide the primary framework. Their straight hydrocarbon chains align closely with adjacent lipids, reducing gaps within the bilayer and lowering baseline permeability. As these lipids accumulate through remodeling cycles, the membrane becomes more resistant to uncontrolled ion and proton movement. This strengthens gradient maintenance in both cellular and mitochondrial membranes, directly affecting transport efficiency and energy capture. The increased packing also stabilizes the physical platform on which receptors and enzymes operate, reducing variability in how they respond to input.

Monounsaturated fatty acids introduce a controlled degree of flexibility into this framework. The presence of a single double bond creates a consistent bend that prevents excessive rigidity without disrupting overall organization. This allows membranes to retain the ability to accommodate protein conformational changes and lateral movement required for signaling. When incorporated alongside saturated lipids, monounsaturated fatty acids define a functional range of fluidity where receptors can cluster, separate, and reassemble without losing structural coherence.

The interaction between these two classes determines membrane behavior under varying conditions. Saturated lipids anchor the structure, while monounsaturated lipids modulate spacing to maintain functional mobility. When this balance is achieved, membranes resist deformation under mechanical stress and maintain consistent permeability across temperature changes. This stability allows cellular processes to operate within defined constraints rather than adapting continuously to fluctuating structural conditions.

Cholesterol integrates into this rebuilt environment as a regulator rather than a compensator. Within a membrane composed of stable substrates, cholesterol fine-tunes local packing by preventing excessive fluidity and limiting rigid crystallization. This maintains uniformity across regions of the membrane, supporting the formation of organized domains where signaling proteins can localize and interact. Without a stable base of saturated and monounsaturated lipids, cholesterol cannot perform this role effectively, and its distribution becomes uneven.

Mitochondrial membranes reflect the same principles. As saturated and monounsaturated lipids replace more permeable structures, the inner membrane regains its ability to confine the proton gradient generated by electron transport. Reduced leakage increases the proportion of energy captured as ATP, lowering the need for compensatory increases in substrate oxidation. This stabilizes cellular energy supply and supports processes that depend on consistent ATP availability.

Receptor function improves as the surrounding lipid environment becomes more consistent. Insulin receptors, ion channels, and other membrane proteins rely on a stable platform to undergo conformational changes and interact with downstream components. When the bilayer provides uniform mechanical resistance and controlled fluidity, these proteins operate with greater precision. Signal initiation, amplification, and termination align more closely with input, reducing the variability that characterizes unstable membranes.

Remodeling cycles gradually embed this balance across tissues. Each cycle replaces a portion of existing lipids with those available in circulation. Sustained availability of saturated and monounsaturated substrates ensures that new membrane segments reflect the desired structural properties. Over time, variability between tissues decreases as composition converges toward a common baseline that supports coordinated function.

Resistance to oxidative damage increases as these lipids become predominant. With fewer highly reactive double bonds, the likelihood of chain reactions decreases, allowing membranes to maintain integrity under metabolic and environmental stress. Repair systems operate more effectively because the rate of damage is reduced, reinforcing the stability achieved through composition.

Saturated and monounsaturated rebuilding therefore establishes the mechanical conditions required for consistent cellular behavior. By providing a foundation that supports tight packing and controlled flexibility, these lipids allow membranes to maintain gradients, organize signaling domains, and resist degradation. The system regains coherence as each remodeling cycle integrates these properties, producing a structure that supports efficient and coordinated function across tissues.

Time-Dependent Membrane Replacement

Membrane reconstruction unfolds according to turnover rates that differ across tissues, not according to the timing of any single input. Each membrane is continuously renewed through cycles of degradation and synthesis, where existing phospholipids are broken down and replaced with new ones assembled from circulating substrates. This process operates at a pace defined by cellular activity, metabolic demand, and exposure to stress. When the substrate pool shifts toward stable lipids, the effect is not immediate because existing structures remain in place until they are replaced. Change appears as a gradual transition where newly incorporated lipids alter local properties first, then spread across the membrane as turnover continues.

The replacement process begins at the level of individual phospholipids. Enzymatic pathways remove fatty acids from existing molecules and re-esterify them with those available in circulation. This selective exchange allows the membrane to adjust composition without requiring complete dismantling. As stable substrates become more available, these enzymes incorporate them into new phospholipids, progressively altering the characteristics of the bilayer. The rate of this exchange determines how quickly structural changes manifest within a given tissue.

Turnover varies significantly between cell types. Tissues with high metabolic activity, such as the liver and intestinal epithelium, replace membrane components rapidly due to constant exposure to substrates and environmental inputs. These tissues respond more quickly to changes in lipid availability, showing early shifts in permeability, signaling behavior, and energy handling. In contrast, tissues with slower turnover, such as neural structures and long-lived cells, require extended periods of consistent input to achieve comparable changes. Their membranes retain previous composition longer, delaying full reconstruction.

Mitochondrial membranes follow a similar pattern but are influenced by both lipid turnover and organelle dynamics. Fusion and fission processes redistribute membrane components across the mitochondrial network, allowing localized improvements to spread over time. As new lipids are incorporated into individual mitochondria, these dynamics facilitate the gradual normalization of membrane properties across the entire population.

The cumulative nature of replacement defines the trajectory of stabilization. Early changes may be subtle, affecting only small regions of the membrane or specific cellular functions. As successive cycles incorporate stable lipids, these regions expand, and the overall behavior of the membrane shifts. Gradients become easier to maintain, receptor function becomes more consistent, and energy production stabilizes. These improvements do not occur in isolation but build upon one another as the proportion of stable structure increases.

External conditions influence the pace of this process. Continued exposure to unstable or oxidized lipids slows progress by reintroducing components that counteract reconstruction. Conversely, maintaining a consistent supply of stable substrates allows each cycle to contribute to the same direction of change, accelerating convergence toward a stable configuration.

Energy availability also affects turnover. Membrane synthesis, repair, and remodeling require ATP. When mitochondrial efficiency improves, these processes can proceed at a rate that supports effective replacement. When energy is limited, turnover slows, prolonging the presence of unstable structures.

Time-dependent replacement therefore governs how structural changes propagate through the system. The body does not rebuild membranes instantly but through continuous, incremental updates that reflect the current substrate environment. As stable lipids are incorporated across successive cycles, the membrane transitions from a variable and permeable state to one that maintains consistent packing, controlled exchange, and reliable signaling behavior across tissues.

Restoring Electrical and Signaling Stability

Electrical behavior in biological systems is defined by how well membranes separate charge and control ion movement. Every gradient across a membrane represents stored potential that can be used to drive transport, generate signals, or sustain cellular work. When membrane structure becomes inconsistent, this separation weakens. Ions cross more freely, gradients dissipate, and the baseline electrical state of the cell becomes unstable. Restoring stability requires rebuilding membranes that can maintain charge separation with minimal leakage, allowing electrical properties to remain consistent across time and across tissues.

Ion channels and transporters depend on this environment to function correctly. These proteins do not generate gradients on their own. They regulate the movement of ions according to the conditions established by the membrane. When permeability increases, passive ion flow competes with controlled transport, forcing channels and pumps to work continuously to maintain balance. This increases energy demand and reduces the precision of electrical signaling. As membrane integrity improves, passive leakage decreases, and transport systems regain the ability to establish and maintain gradients with less effort, stabilizing the electrical baseline of the cell.

Membrane potential becomes more consistent as structural integrity is restored. The difference in charge between the inside and outside of the cell depends on selective permeability and active transport. When the membrane supports tight packing and controlled ion movement, this potential remains stable, providing a reliable platform for signaling events. Fluctuations decrease, and the cell can respond to inputs without interference from background instability.

Receptor function is directly influenced by these electrical conditions. Many signaling processes depend on changes in membrane potential or on the local ionic environment. When the baseline is unstable, receptor activation becomes less predictable, and downstream signaling pathways receive inconsistent input. Stabilizing the membrane restores the conditions required for receptors to respond proportionally to stimuli, improving the clarity of signal transmission.

Synaptic and neuronal signaling rely heavily on these principles. Transmission of electrical impulses depends on rapid, controlled changes in membrane potential. When membranes cannot maintain consistent gradients, signal propagation becomes irregular. This affects timing, amplitude, and coordination of neural activity. As membrane properties normalize, conduction becomes more reliable, and communication between cells regains precision.

Mitochondrial membranes contribute to electrical stability through their role in maintaining proton gradients. These gradients represent a form of electrical potential that drives ATP synthesis. When leakage is reduced, the gradient remains stable, supporting consistent energy production. This ensures that energy-dependent signaling processes have a reliable supply of ATP, further stabilizing cellular behavior.

Signal termination improves as stability returns. In a stable membrane, channels close, receptors disengage, and gradients are restored to baseline conditions in a controlled manner. When structure is inconsistent, these processes are delayed or incomplete, leading to prolonged or overlapping signals. Restoring membrane integrity allows signals to begin and end within defined time frames, reducing interference between pathways.

Coordination across tissues depends on the consistency of these electrical properties. When membranes across different cell types maintain similar baseline conditions, signals transmitted through neural and endocrine systems produce aligned responses. Variability decreases, and the system operates with greater coherence.

Restoring electrical and signaling stability therefore depends on rebuilding membranes that can maintain charge separation, regulate ion movement, and support predictable receptor behavior. As leakage is reduced and gradients are preserved, the system regains the ability to process and transmit signals with precision, allowing coordinated function to emerge from a stable structural foundation.

Chapter 22

Restoring Signaling Precision

Signaling precision depends on the ability of the membrane to present a consistent environment in which receptors detect input, assemble into functional complexes, and terminate activity within defined timeframes. Precision is not created at the level of the signal itself. It emerges from the structural conditions that determine how that signal is interpreted. When membrane composition varies, identical inputs produce different outputs across cells and tissues. Restoring precision therefore requires rebuilding a membrane environment that enforces uniform rules for activation, amplification, and termination.

Receptor activation depends on controlled proximity. Ligand binding increases the likelihood that receptors interact with one another and initiate signaling, but this process requires a balance between mobility and constraint. If the membrane is too rigid, receptors cannot move into position efficiently, reducing activation. If too fluid, receptors encounter one another randomly and outside of organized domains, producing unstable or incomplete signals. A membrane composed of stable lipids maintains a range of fluidity where receptors can cluster within defined regions, allowing activation to occur only when input reaches a sufficient threshold.

Microdomain organization governs where signaling occurs. Specific lipids and proteins segregate into regions that concentrate receptors and downstream components. These domains provide a controlled environment for signal propagation, ensuring that interactions occur in a coordinated sequence. When membrane structure is inconsistent, these domains become unstable, and signaling components disperse. This disrupts the sequence of interactions required for precise output. As composition stabilizes, domains reform, and signaling pathways regain spatial organization.

Signal amplification depends on the integrity of these domains. Once activated, receptors recruit additional proteins to propagate the signal. This process requires stable anchoring points within the membrane. When the surrounding lipid environment supports consistent packing, these interactions proceed efficiently, producing a response that reflects the original input. In unstable membranes, amplification becomes uneven, with some signals expanding excessively and others failing to propagate.

Termination defines the boundary of signaling events. Precision requires that signals end once their function is complete. This involves dissociation of receptor complexes, deactivation of downstream components, and restoration of baseline conditions. Membrane structure influences how quickly and reliably these processes occur. Increased permeability and disorganization prolong interactions and delay termination, leading to overlapping signals. Restoring structural integrity allows signaling complexes to disassemble in a controlled manner, re-establishing clear boundaries between events.

Cross-talk between pathways is reduced as precision improves. In unstable membranes, overlapping signals interfere with one another because components are not confined to specific regions. This creates noise within the system, where unrelated pathways influence each other. Organized domains limit these interactions, allowing pathways to operate independently while still integrating at higher levels when required.

Energy availability supports signaling precision. Activation, propagation, and termination all require ATP. When mitochondrial efficiency improves and gradients are maintained, energy supply becomes consistent, allowing signaling processes to proceed without interruption. This reduces variability in response and supports the timing required for coordinated function.

System-wide coordination emerges from local precision. When individual cells interpret signals consistently, tissues respond in a unified manner. Hormonal inputs produce aligned effects, neural signals propagate with predictable timing, and immune responses remain proportional to input. This alignment depends on the convergence of membrane properties across tissues, which is achieved through sustained remodeling under stable conditions.

Restoring signaling precision therefore involves rebuilding the structural environment that governs how signals are processed. By establishing membranes that support controlled receptor movement, organized domains, and reliable termination, the system regains the ability to translate input into proportional and coordinated output. The improvement is not driven by stronger signals but by a framework that ensures signals are interpreted accurately at every stage.

Re-establishing Receptor Environments

Receptor function is determined less by the presence of the receptor and more by the membrane environment that surrounds it. Every receptor operates within a localized lipid field that defines its mobility, orientation, and ability to interact with other proteins. When this environment becomes inconsistent, the receptor remains intact but loses the conditions required to translate binding into a controlled signal. Re-establishing receptor environments means restoring the physical constraints that allow receptors to activate, propagate signals, and disengage in a predictable manner.

The first requirement is controlled lateral movement. Receptors must be able to move within the plane of the membrane to encounter other receptors and signaling partners, but that movement must occur within defined limits. A membrane composed of stable lipids provides resistance that prevents random diffusion while still allowing directed interactions. This balance ensures that clustering occurs only when ligand binding increases the probability of interaction, preserving threshold-dependent activation.

Local packing density determines receptor conformation. Many receptors undergo structural changes when activated, and these changes depend on the mechanical properties of the surrounding lipids. When packing is too loose, the receptor lacks the resistance needed to stabilize its active configuration. When too tight, conformational transitions are restricted. Reintroducing a lipid environment with consistent packing allows receptors to shift between states in response to input rather than being constrained or destabilized by the membrane itself.

Microdomain formation provides spatial organization for signaling. Specific lipid compositions create regions where receptors and downstream components concentrate. These domains act as platforms that bring together the elements required for signal propagation. When membrane composition supports domain stability, receptors localize to these regions, increasing the efficiency and specificity of their interactions. Without this organization, signaling components remain dispersed, and the sequence of interactions required for precise output is disrupted.

Electrical conditions within the membrane influence receptor sensitivity. Ion gradients and local charge distribution affect how receptors respond to ligands and how downstream signaling pathways are initiated. Increased permeability alters these conditions, reducing the consistency of receptor activation. Restoring membrane integrity stabilizes these gradients, providing a uniform electrical environment that supports predictable receptor behavior.

Protein-lipid interactions define receptor anchoring. Many receptors interact directly with specific lipids that stabilize their position and orientation within the membrane. When these lipids are replaced by structures that do not support these interactions, receptors become less stable and more prone to irregular movement. Reintroducing lipids that support these interactions restores anchoring, allowing receptors to maintain proper alignment with signaling partners.

Termination of signaling depends on the ability to separate receptor complexes after activation. This requires a membrane environment that allows controlled disassembly without prolonging interactions. When structure is restored, receptors disengage from one another and from associated proteins in a timely manner, preventing overlap between signaling events.

Distribution of receptors across tissues becomes more consistent as environments stabilize. Differences in membrane composition between cell types decrease, allowing receptors to respond similarly to the same input. This reduces variability in system-wide responses and improves coordination between tissues.

Energy availability supports all aspects of receptor function. ATP-dependent processes maintain gradients, facilitate protein interactions, and drive the recycling of receptors after activation. When mitochondrial efficiency improves, these processes operate without interruption, reinforcing the stability of receptor environments.

Re-establishing receptor environments therefore involves reconstructing the lipid context in which receptors operate. By restoring controlled mobility, consistent packing, organized domains, and stable electrical conditions, the membrane provides the framework required for receptors to function with precision. The result is not an increase in receptor number or signal strength, but a restoration of the conditions that allow existing receptors to produce accurate and proportional responses to input.

Normalizing Hormone Response

Hormonal signaling depends on the ability of tissues to interpret circulating signals in a consistent and proportional manner. Hormones are distributed system-wide, but their effects are determined locally at the membrane where receptors detect and translate those signals into intracellular actions. When membrane structure varies across tissues, the same hormone concentration produces different responses, creating a mismatch between signal and outcome. Normalizing hormone response requires restoring a membrane environment that allows receptors to operate under uniform conditions, so that input is translated into output with consistent magnitude and timing.

Receptor sensitivity is defined by the physical properties of the surrounding lipids. Hormone receptors rely on controlled fluidity and stable packing to transition between inactive and active states. When membranes become too permeable or disorganized, these transitions lose precision. Some receptors fail to activate efficiently, while others remain active longer than intended. Re-establishing a balanced lipid environment restores the mechanical constraints needed for receptors to respond proportionally to hormone binding, aligning activation with signal strength.

Signal propagation depends on the assembly of downstream components within organized membrane regions. Hormone binding initiates a sequence of interactions that amplify the signal and produce a cellular response. This sequence requires spatial organization so that proteins encounter each other in a defined order. When membrane domains are unstable, these interactions become inconsistent, and the signal either weakens or spreads beyond its intended scope. As membrane composition stabilizes, these domains reform, allowing signaling pathways to proceed with predictable efficiency.

Termination of hormonal signaling defines the boundary of response. Hormone action must cease once the required effect is achieved to prevent overlap with subsequent signals. Membrane structure influences how quickly receptor complexes disassemble and how effectively downstream pathways return to baseline. Increased permeability and disorganization prolong signaling, creating a state where responses overlap and interfere with one another. Restoring structural integrity allows signals to terminate within defined timeframes, preventing accumulation of activity.

Transport of hormones and secondary messengers is also affected by membrane conditions. Many signaling molecules must cross membranes or move within them to reach their targets. When permeability is altered, this movement becomes less controlled, affecting both the speed and distribution of signaling components. Stabilizing membrane structure ensures that transport occurs through regulated pathways rather than through uncontrolled diffusion, preserving the specificity of hormonal effects.

Energy availability supports the entire signaling process. Hormone response requires ATP for receptor recycling, phosphorylation events, and maintenance of ion gradients. When mitochondrial membranes regain the ability to contain proton gradients, ATP production stabilizes, providing a consistent energy supply for signaling. This reduces variability in response and supports the timing required for coordinated hormone action.

Inter-tissue coordination improves as responses normalize. When membranes across different tissues converge toward similar structural properties, receptors interpret signals in a more uniform manner. Hormones that regulate metabolism, growth, and stress produce aligned effects, allowing the system to respond as a cohesive unit rather than as a collection of independently behaving compartments.

Feedback systems regain effectiveness under these conditions. Hormonal regulation relies on feedback loops that adjust signal output based on response. When responses are inconsistent, feedback signals become distorted, leading to over- or under-correction. As receptor environments stabilize, feedback loops operate with greater accuracy, maintaining hormone levels within ranges that produce appropriate responses.

Normalizing hormone response therefore involves restoring the structural conditions that govern how signals are interpreted at the membrane level. By rebuilding a consistent lipid environment, receptors regain the ability to activate, propagate, and terminate signals in alignment with input. The system does not require stronger signals but a stable framework that allows existing signals to produce accurate and coordinated effects across tissues.

Stabilizing Inflammatory Signaling

Inflammatory signaling depends on controlled initiation, spatial confinement, and timely termination. These conditions are set at the membrane, where substrate availability determines which mediators can be produced, and where receptor organization determines how signals are amplified and resolved. When membrane composition becomes inconsistent, both the generation and interpretation of inflammatory signals drift. Stabilization requires re-establishing a substrate environment and structural context that limit unnecessary initiation and support completion once signaling has begun.

Initiation is governed by the availability of fatty acid precursors embedded within the membrane. Enzymatic release of these substrates produces signaling molecules that drive inflammation. When the membrane is enriched with highly reactive and easily mobilized lipids, the threshold for initiation decreases, allowing signaling to begin with minimal stimulus. As composition shifts toward more stable lipids, the rate of spontaneous or low-threshold activation declines. This does not eliminate inflammatory capacity. It restores the requirement for a defined trigger before signaling begins.

Amplification depends on receptor clustering within organized domains. Once mediators are produced, they bind to receptors that initiate cascades affecting neighboring cells. This process requires spatial coordination so that signals are contained and directed. In unstable membranes, receptors are dispersed or form transient clusters that amplify signals unevenly. Some regions over-respond, while others fail to propagate the signal. Rebuilding membrane organization allows receptors to localize within defined regions, producing amplification that reflects the original input rather than random variability.

Termination is the critical step that defines whether inflammation resolves or persists. Resolution pathways depend on the generation of mediators that actively suppress signaling and restore baseline conditions. These pathways require specific substrates and a membrane environment that supports their production. When substrate availability is limited or membrane structure disrupts enzymatic activity, termination signals are insufficient. The response continues beyond its intended duration, creating a state of persistent activation. Stabilization involves ensuring that both the substrates and structural conditions required for resolution are present, allowing signaling to complete its cycle.

Membrane permeability influences the spread of inflammatory signals. Increased permeability allows mediators and ions to move beyond their intended range, expanding the area of activation. This reduces the ability to localize responses and increases the likelihood of system-wide effects from a localized trigger. As membrane integrity improves, diffusion becomes more controlled, and signaling remains confined to appropriate regions.

Oxidative processes interact with inflammatory signaling at multiple levels. Reactive species generated during inflammation can further damage membrane lipids, increasing susceptibility to additional signaling events. This creates a feedback loop where inflammation promotes conditions that sustain itself. Reducing oxidative load and stabilizing membrane composition interrupts this cycle, limiting the propagation of damage and allowing resolution mechanisms to function effectively.

Energy availability supports both activation and termination. Inflammatory signaling requires ATP for mediator synthesis, receptor activity, and cellular responses. Resolution processes also depend on energy to restore baseline conditions and repair damaged structures. When mitochondrial efficiency improves, the system can complete the full signaling cycle rather than remaining in a prolonged activated state due to insufficient energy for termination.

Intercellular coordination improves as signaling stabilizes. Immune cells communicate through mediators that depend on consistent interpretation across tissues. When membrane conditions align, these signals produce coordinated responses that are proportional and localized. Variability decreases, and the immune system operates with greater precision.

Stabilizing inflammatory signaling therefore involves controlling both the substrates that initiate the response and the structural conditions that govern its progression. By restoring membrane composition and organization, the system regains the ability to initiate inflammation when required, amplify it within defined boundaries, and terminate it once its function is complete. The result is a signaling process that operates within controlled limits rather than persisting as an unresolved and self-reinforcing state.

Improving System Coherence

System coherence emerges when tissues interpret inputs under the same structural conditions and produce aligned outputs over time. It is not created by increasing signal strength or adding regulatory layers. It depends on restoring a shared membrane baseline so that transport, signaling, and energy production follow the same rules across organs. When membranes differ in composition and behavior, each tissue processes identical inputs in a different way, and coordination breaks down. Improving coherence requires reducing that variability until responses converge.

Signal interpretation becomes uniform as receptor environments stabilize. Hormones, neurotransmitters, and local mediators arrive with defined concentration and timing, but their effects depend on receptor behavior within each tissue. When membrane composition converges, receptor clustering, activation thresholds, and termination kinetics align. The same input produces a similar response profile across cells, reducing conflicting outputs. This allows endocrine and neural signals to coordinate rather than compete.

Transport regains consistency when permeability and gradient control are restored. Substrate movement depends on maintained differences in concentration and charge. In unstable membranes, passive leakage competes with regulated transport, creating uneven distribution. As membranes rebuild with tighter packing and controlled fluidity, gradients hold with less energy, and transporters operate under predictable conditions. Nutrients and ions are delivered according to demand rather than drifting toward regions of least resistance.

Energy distribution stabilizes as mitochondrial membranes regain containment. Efficient proton gradients increase ATP yield per unit of substrate, reducing the need for compensatory overconsumption. When energy production becomes consistent across tissues, processes that depend on ATP operate with less variability. This supports synchronized function, as cells no longer experience alternating states of surplus and deficit that distort signaling and transport.

Temporal alignment improves when activation and termination occur within defined windows. Many physiological processes depend on timing, including hormone pulses, neural firing patterns, and immune responses.

Membrane instability prolongs or shortens these windows unpredictably. As structural integrity returns, signals begin and end within consistent durations, allowing processes to sequence correctly rather than overlap or interfere with one another.

Feedback systems regain accuracy under coherent conditions. Regulatory loops depend on consistent relationships between input and output. When responses vary between tissues, feedback signals misrepresent the state of the system, leading to overcorrection or persistent imbalance. With aligned membrane behavior, outputs reflect inputs more reliably, and feedback loops adjust signals with greater precision.

Inter-tissue communication becomes more effective as variability decreases. Signals transmitted through blood or neural pathways are interpreted similarly across different organs, allowing coordinated adjustments to changing conditions. The system operates as an integrated network rather than as independent compartments responding in isolation.

Remodeling cycles reinforce coherence when the substrate pool supports stable composition. Each cycle reduces variability by replacing divergent structures with a common set of lipid properties. Over time, differences between tissues narrow, and the system approaches a unified baseline. This does not eliminate specialization, but it ensures that specialized functions operate within a consistent structural framework.

Energy demand for maintenance decreases as coherence improves. Fewer resources are required to correct imbalances caused by inconsistent signaling or transport. This allows the system to allocate energy toward productive processes rather than continuous compensation, further stabilizing function.

Improving system coherence therefore involves converging membrane properties across tissues so that inputs are processed under shared conditions. As variability in structure declines, signaling, transport, and energy production align, allowing the body to function as a coordinated system with predictable and efficient responses to internal and external demands.

Chapter 23

Rebuilding Mitochondrial Efficiency

Mitochondrial efficiency is defined by how effectively the inner membrane can convert substrate oxidation into a contained proton gradient and then into ATP. The machinery of the electron transport chain remains functional across a wide range of conditions, but its output depends on the integrity of the membrane that surrounds it. When the membrane allows uncontrolled proton movement or fails to maintain the organization of its protein complexes, energy is lost during conversion. Rebuilding efficiency therefore centers on restoring the structural conditions that allow the gradient to be generated, contained, and used with minimal loss.

The inner membrane must re-establish low permeability. Proton containment is the core requirement for efficient ATP production. As stable lipids replace more permissive structures, the bilayer becomes less susceptible to uncontrolled proton flow. This reduces leakage and increases the proportion of the gradient that is available for ATP synthesis. The change does not alter the capacity of the electron transport chain itself. It improves how effectively that capacity is translated into usable energy.

Cardiolipin plays a central role in organizing the electron transport chain. This phospholipid anchors complexes within the membrane and maintains their spatial relationship, allowing electrons to move through the chain in a controlled sequence. When cardiolipin composition is altered or damaged, these relationships become unstable, and electron flow becomes less efficient. Rebuilding membrane integrity supports the proper structure of cardiolipin, restoring the alignment of complexes and reducing the likelihood of electron escape.

Electron leakage decreases as structural organization improves. When electrons move through the chain efficiently, fewer deviate from their intended path to form reactive species. This reduces oxidative stress within the mitochondrion and limits damage to lipids, proteins, and mitochondrial DNA. Lower oxidative load further supports membrane stability, reinforcing the conditions required for efficient energy production.

ATP synthase operates more effectively within a stable gradient. This enzyme depends on a consistent flow of protons through its channel to drive the conversion of ADP to ATP. When the gradient is weakened by leakage, the rate of ATP production declines, and the system compensates by increasing substrate oxidation. As membrane integrity improves and the gradient strengthens, ATP synthase can operate at a higher efficiency, reducing the need for compensatory increases in input.

Mitochondrial dynamics contribute to the rebuilding process. Fusion allows mitochondria with improved membrane properties to share components with others, spreading functional improvements across the network. Fission removes segments that remain damaged or inefficient, allowing them to be targeted for degradation. These processes depend on both membrane integrity and energy availability, and they become more effective as conditions stabilize.

Energy availability improves as efficiency increases. With less energy lost through proton leakage and reactive species formation, a greater proportion of substrate oxidation is converted into ATP. This stabilizes cellular energy supply, supporting processes that depend on consistent ATP levels, including transport, signaling, and repair.

Substrate utilization becomes more balanced under these conditions. When mitochondria operate efficiently, the system does not require excessive input to maintain output. This reduces strain on metabolic pathways and limits the accumulation of intermediate products that can disrupt cellular function. The relationship between substrate availability and energy production becomes more proportional.

Repair mechanisms within the mitochondrion operate more effectively as oxidative damage decreases. Enzymes responsible for maintaining mitochondrial DNA and protein integrity require energy and a stable environment. As efficiency improves, these systems can keep pace with damage, preserving function over time.

Rebuilding mitochondrial efficiency therefore involves restoring the structural integrity of the inner membrane so that electron transport, proton gradient formation, and ATP synthesis operate within controlled conditions. The machinery remains present throughout, but its output becomes aligned with input only when the membrane provides the containment and organization required for efficient energy conversion.

Cardiolipin Restoration

Cardiolipin defines the inner mitochondrial membrane as a functional surface rather than a simple barrier. It anchors electron transport complexes, stabilizes their orientation, and maintains the curvature required for dense packing of cristae. When cardiolipin is intact and correctly composed, the membrane holds these complexes in close proximity, allowing electrons to move through the chain with minimal deviation. When it is depleted, oxidized, or remodeled into less stable forms, this organization breaks down. Restoration therefore focuses on rebuilding both the quantity and structural integrity of cardiolipin so that the membrane can support controlled energy conversion.

Synthesis begins with the availability of appropriate lipid substrates and sufficient energy. Cardiolipin is assembled within the inner membrane using precursor phospholipids that reflect the circulating lipid pool. When stable fatty acids dominate, newly synthesized cardiolipin forms with acyl chains that support tight packing and resistance to deformation. This improves its ability to anchor protein complexes and maintain the local membrane environment required for efficient electron transfer.

Remodeling refines cardiolipin composition after initial synthesis. Enzymatic processes replace fatty acyl chains to produce a more uniform structure that matches the functional requirements of the mitochondrion. When the substrate pool contains unstable or highly oxidizable lipids, remodeling incorporates these components, reducing cardiolipin stability. Shifting the available substrates allows remodeling to produce a more consistent and durable form, improving its ability to maintain membrane organization.

Oxidative damage represents a primary source of cardiolipin dysfunction. Located adjacent to the electron transport chain, cardiolipin is exposed to reactive species generated during electron transfer. When these species interact with its acyl chains, they alter its structure and reduce its ability to bind and stabilize protein complexes. Damaged cardiolipin disrupts electron flow, increasing leakage and further oxidative stress. Reducing oxidative load and limiting the presence of highly susceptible lipids lowers the rate of this damage, allowing restoration processes to outpace degradation.

Cristae structure depends on cardiolipin integrity. The folds of the inner membrane increase surface area and create compartments that concentrate electron transport components. Cardiolipin contributes to the curvature and stability of these structures. When its composition is compromised, cristae become less defined, reducing the efficiency of energy production. Restoration of cardiolipin supports the reformation of these structures, improving the spatial organization of the electron transport chain.

Protein interactions are stabilized as cardiolipin integrity improves. Many components of the electron transport chain require direct interaction with cardiolipin to maintain their conformation and activity. When this interaction is disrupted, complexes become less efficient and more prone to releasing electrons prematurely. Re-establishing cardiolipin structure restores these interactions, reducing electron leakage and improving the consistency of energy conversion.

Mitochondrial dynamics assist in distributing restored cardiolipin. Fusion events allow mitochondria with improved membrane composition to share lipids and proteins, spreading stability across the network. Fission isolates regions that remain damaged, enabling their removal through quality control processes. These dynamics accelerate the normalization of cardiolipin across the mitochondrial population.

Energy production improves as cardiolipin is restored. With better organization of electron transport complexes and reduced proton leakage, a greater proportion of substrate oxidation is converted into ATP. This stabilizes cellular energy supply and reduces the need for compensatory increases in metabolic throughput.

Repair processes within the mitochondrion become more effective as oxidative damage decreases and cardiolipin composition stabilizes. Enzymes responsible for maintaining mitochondrial components operate within a more controlled environment, allowing them to preserve function over time.

Cardiolipin restoration therefore re-establishes the structural foundation of the inner mitochondrial membrane. By rebuilding its composition and protecting it from ongoing damage, the membrane regains its ability to organize electron transport, contain the proton gradient, and support efficient ATP production. The improvement in mitochondrial function follows directly from the restoration of this lipid framework rather than from changes in the protein machinery itself.

Reducing Electron Leak and ROS Production

Electron leak occurs when electrons deviate from their intended path through the electron transport chain and react prematurely with oxygen. This is not a failure of the chain itself but a consequence of structural conditions that disrupt controlled transfer. The inner mitochondrial membrane must maintain both the spatial organization of complexes and the confinement of charge to ensure that electrons move stepwise through defined carriers. When this organization weakens, electrons escape, forming reactive species that do not contribute to ATP production and instead propagate damage within the membrane.

The stability of electron flow depends on how closely the complexes are arranged. Cardiolipin anchors these complexes and maintains their alignment, allowing electrons to pass efficiently between them. When cardiolipin structure is compromised, the distance and orientation between complexes change, increasing the probability that electrons will not reach their intended destination. Restoring membrane composition re-establishes these relationships, reducing the likelihood of premature electron transfer to oxygen.

Proton gradient containment influences electron behavior. A stable gradient creates back-pressure that regulates the rate of electron transport. When protons leak across the membrane, this pressure decreases, and electron flow accelerates in an uncontrolled manner. This increases the chance of electrons escaping the chain. By reducing membrane permeability and restoring gradient containment, electron flow becomes more controlled, lowering the rate of leakage.

Lipid composition determines susceptibility to secondary reactions once reactive species are formed. Membranes rich in highly unsaturated fatty acids provide multiple sites for these species to initiate chain reactions. As stable lipids replace these structures, the number of reactive targets decreases, limiting the propagation of damage even when small amounts of reactive species are produced.

Antioxidant systems within the mitochondrion intercept reactive intermediates before they can interact with surrounding lipids. These systems rely on both availability of antioxidant molecules and proper localization within the membrane. When oxidative load is reduced and membrane organization improves, these defenses can neutralize reactive species more effectively, preventing accumulation.

Electron input must remain matched to the capacity of the transport chain. Excess substrate delivery increases the rate of electron donation, which can overwhelm the system when structural conditions are suboptimal. As mitochondrial efficiency improves, electron flow aligns more closely with the capacity for controlled transfer, reducing the pressure that leads to leakage.

Mitochondrial dynamics contribute to reducing electron leak by maintaining a population of functional organelles. Fusion allows mitochondria with stable membranes to share components, improving overall performance. Fission isolates regions where electron leak remains high, enabling their removal through quality control mechanisms. This maintains a network that operates with reduced variability in electron transport.

Energy production becomes more efficient as electron leak decreases. Fewer electrons are lost to reactive pathways, and a greater proportion contributes to proton gradient formation and ATP synthesis. This reduces the need for compensatory increases in substrate oxidation and lowers the overall oxidative burden on the system.

Reducing electron leak and reactive species production therefore depends on restoring the structural integrity of the inner mitochondrial membrane and aligning electron flow with its capacity. By improving complex organization, maintaining gradient containment, and limiting susceptible substrates, the system reduces the frequency and impact of electron deviation. The result is a more efficient conversion of substrate energy into ATP and a lower rate of membrane damage from reactive intermediates.

Re-establishing Gradient Integrity

The proton gradient across the inner mitochondrial membrane represents stored energy in its most usable form. Electron transport builds this gradient by moving protons into the intermembrane space, creating both a concentration difference and an electrical potential. ATP synthesis depends on forcing those protons back through a controlled pathway. When the membrane holds the gradient tightly, the flow is directed through ATP synthase and energy is captured efficiently. When containment weakens, protons return through the bilayer or through non-specific pathways, and the stored potential dissipates without producing work. Re-establishing gradient integrity means restoring the membrane conditions that prevent this uncontrolled return.

Permeability is the primary variable. The inner membrane must resist proton movement except through defined channels. This resistance is determined by lipid packing density and the absence of structural defects that allow charge to bypass ATP synthase. As stable lipids replace more permissive structures, the bilayer becomes less conductive to proton flow, and leakage declines. Even small reductions in permeability have large effects on gradient stability because the system operates continuously. Lower leakage allows the gradient to build and persist with less input from electron transport.

Electrical properties of the membrane contribute to gradient maintenance. The separation of charge across the bilayer creates an electrical field that influences how protons move. A stable membrane maintains this field without fluctuations caused by uncontrolled ion movement. When permeability increases, other ions cross more freely, dissipating the electrical component of the gradient. Restoring structural integrity limits this movement, preserving both the chemical and electrical components that together define the gradient.

The organization of the electron transport chain affects how efficiently the gradient is generated. Complexes must be positioned so that electron flow is continuous and proton pumping occurs in a coordinated manner. Cardiolipin stabilizes this arrangement, ensuring that protons are moved into the intermembrane space at a rate that matches the capacity of the membrane to contain them. When this organization is restored, gradient formation becomes more consistent, reducing fluctuations that would otherwise weaken overall integrity.

ATP synthase depends on a stable gradient to operate efficiently. This enzyme converts the potential energy stored in the gradient into chemical energy in the form of ATP. When the gradient is inconsistent, the flow of protons through ATP synthase becomes irregular, reducing the rate and efficiency of ATP production. As gradient integrity improves, proton flow becomes steady and directed, allowing ATP synthesis to proceed at a rate that reflects the actual capacity of the system.

Substrate oxidation becomes more efficient when gradient integrity is maintained. With less energy lost to leakage, the system does not require excessive input to sustain ATP production. This reduces the burden on metabolic pathways and lowers the generation of reactive species associated with high throughput conditions. The relationship between substrate input and energy output becomes more proportional.

Mitochondrial dynamics support gradient restoration by distributing stable membrane components across the network. Fusion events allow regions with improved integrity to influence others, while fission isolates areas where leakage persists. This process gradually increases the proportion of mitochondria capable of maintaining strong gradients.

Energy-dependent maintenance processes benefit from improved gradient integrity. Ion pumps, transport systems, and repair mechanisms rely on consistent ATP availability. As ATP production stabilizes, these processes operate more effectively, reinforcing the structural conditions that support gradient maintenance.

Re-establishing gradient integrity therefore involves restoring the physical properties of the inner mitochondrial membrane so that protons are confined and directed through controlled pathways. By reducing permeability, preserving electrical stability, and maintaining the organization of electron transport complexes, the system rebuilds the conditions required for efficient energy conversion. The gradient becomes a reliable store of potential energy rather than a transient state that dissipates before it can be used.

Recovering Energy Consistency

Energy consistency is defined by the ability to produce ATP at a stable rate under varying conditions without requiring continuous compensation. The system does not fail because it cannot generate energy. It fails because production becomes variable, forcing constant adjustment in substrate use, signaling intensity, and cellular behavior. This variability originates at the membrane level, where inefficiency in gradient containment and electron transport introduces fluctuations in output. Recovering consistency requires restoring the structural conditions that allow energy production to proceed at a predictable rate.

Mitochondrial membranes must maintain stable gradients over time. When proton leakage is reduced and electron flow is controlled, the gradient does not collapse between cycles of ATP synthesis. This allows ATP production to proceed continuously rather than in bursts followed by depletion. The result is a steady supply of energy that supports processes requiring constant input, such as ion transport and protein turnover.

Substrate utilization becomes aligned with demand. In an unstable system, increased leakage forces higher substrate oxidation to maintain output, creating periods of excess input followed by relative shortage. As efficiency improves, the amount of substrate required to sustain ATP production decreases, allowing intake and utilization to remain proportional. This reduces fluctuations in circulating substrates and stabilizes metabolic pathways.

Signal-dependent energy demand is met more effectively under consistent conditions. Cellular signaling processes require ATP for activation, propagation, and termination. When energy supply fluctuates, signaling becomes inconsistent, with some pathways receiving sufficient support while others do not. Stabilizing ATP production allows signaling processes to proceed without interruption, improving coordination within and between cells.

Ion gradients are maintained with less effort. Pumps that regulate sodium, potassium, calcium, and other ions depend on ATP to sustain differences across membranes. When ATP availability is stable, these gradients remain constant, supporting electrical stability and transport processes. This reduces the need for compensatory activity that would otherwise increase energy demand and introduce variability.

Mitochondrial dynamics reinforce consistency. Fusion distributes functional components across the network, allowing mitochondria with stable membranes to support those that are less efficient. Fission isolates regions that continue to produce inconsistent output, enabling their removal. Over time, this process increases the proportion of mitochondria capable of maintaining steady energy production.

Repair and maintenance processes operate more effectively when energy supply is stable. These processes require continuous ATP input to replace damaged components and maintain structural integrity. Variability in energy production limits their effectiveness, allowing damage to accumulate. As consistency returns, repair mechanisms keep pace with degradation, preserving function.

Hormonal and neural regulation align with energy availability. Many regulatory systems adjust activity based on perceived energy status. When production is inconsistent, these systems receive conflicting signals, leading to over- or under-compensation. Stable ATP production provides a reliable indicator of system state, allowing regulatory pathways to maintain balance without excessive adjustment.

Temporal coordination improves as energy becomes consistent. Processes that depend on timing, such as metabolic transitions and cellular cycles, require predictable energy availability. When ATP supply fluctuates, these processes become irregular, leading to inefficiency and interference between pathways. A stable energy baseline allows these processes to proceed in sequence, improving overall system function.

Recovering energy consistency therefore involves restoring the membrane conditions that allow ATP production to match demand without fluctuation. By reducing leakage, stabilizing electron flow, and aligning substrate use with output, the system re-establishes a steady energy supply. This consistency supports transport, signaling, and repair processes, allowing the body to operate without the need for continuous compensation and adjustment.

PART VII

INTEGRATED SYSTEM RECOVERY

Chapter 24

From Fragmentation to Coordination

Fragmentation develops when tissues operate under different structural conditions and no longer interpret shared inputs in the same way. Each organ continues to receive the same signals, substrates, and regulatory cues, but the membrane environment determines how those inputs are translated into output. When membrane composition diverges across tissues, responses become inconsistent in magnitude, timing, and duration. Coordination is not lost because signals are absent. It is lost because the system no longer shares a common structural framework for interpreting them. Restoring coordination requires convergence back to a uniform membrane baseline that enforces consistent behavior across tissues.

Signal alignment is the first layer to return. Hormonal and neural inputs carry defined information, but their meaning depends on receptor environments within each tissue. When membrane properties stabilize, receptor clustering, activation thresholds, and termination kinetics begin to match across cells. The same input produces a similar response profile regardless of location. This reduces conflicting outputs where one tissue amplifies a signal while another dampens it, allowing signals to propagate through the system without distortion.

Transport coordination follows as gradients become consistent. Movement of substrates, ions, and signaling molecules depends on controlled permeability and maintained differences in concentration. In a fragmented system, these properties vary, creating uneven distribution. Some tissues accumulate substrates while others remain deprived despite adequate supply. As membranes rebuild, permeability decreases and gradients hold more effectively, allowing transport systems to deliver substrates according to demand. Distribution becomes proportional rather than opportunistic.

Energy synchronization emerges as mitochondrial efficiency improves across tissues. When some cells operate under conditions of high leakage and others maintain stronger gradients, energy availability differs between compartments. This creates asynchronous behavior, where processes accelerate in some tissues and slow in others. As membrane integrity converges, ATP production stabilizes system-wide, allowing processes that depend on energy to proceed at similar rates. This alignment reduces interference between pathways that previously operated out of phase.

Temporal coordination becomes possible when signaling and energy supply operate within defined windows. Activation and termination of processes occur in sequence rather than overlapping unpredictably. Hormonal pulses produce effects that rise and fall within expected durations, neural signals propagate with consistent timing, and repair cycles complete without interruption. This sequencing depends on stable membrane conditions that allow signals to begin and end without distortion.

Feedback systems regain coherence as outputs align with inputs. Regulatory loops depend on accurate representation of system state. When tissues respond inconsistently, feedback signals become unreliable, leading to overcorrection or persistent imbalance. With restored structural consistency, outputs reflect inputs more accurately, allowing feedback mechanisms to maintain equilibrium without excessive adjustment.

Inter-system communication becomes more precise. Endocrine, neural, and immune systems exchange information continuously, but their ability to coordinate depends on consistent interpretation of signals. As membrane properties converge, these systems operate with shared rules, allowing signals to produce integrated responses rather than competing or conflicting effects.

Remodeling cycles reinforce coordination over time. Each cycle replaces divergent structures with lipids that support consistent packing and signaling behavior. As this process continues, variability between tissues decreases, and the system approaches a unified structural state. Specialization remains, but it operates within a stable framework that supports coordination.

Energy demand for maintaining balance decreases as fragmentation resolves. Fewer resources are required to compensate for inconsistencies in signaling and transport. This allows the system to allocate energy toward productive functions rather than continuous correction, further stabilizing coordination.

From fragmentation to coordination therefore describes the transition from a system where tissues operate under conflicting structural conditions to one where they share a common membrane baseline. As this baseline is restored, signaling, transport, and energy production align, allowing the body to function as an integrated system with predictable and efficient responses to internal and external inputs.

Reintegration of Metabolic, Immune, and Neural Systems

Metabolic, immune, and neural systems do not operate as independent modules. They share substrates, signals, and structural constraints, and their outputs depend on how consistently those constraints are maintained across tissues. Fragmentation separates their behavior by introducing variability at the membrane level, where each system interprets inputs differently. Reintegration occurs when this variability is reduced and a shared structural baseline is restored, allowing signals to be translated into coordinated responses rather than competing or conflicting actions.

Metabolic signaling provides the substrate context for the other systems. Availability of glucose, fatty acids, and amino acids determines energy status and influences how cells respond to incoming signals. When membrane integrity is restored, transport systems deliver these substrates in proportion to demand, and mitochondrial efficiency converts them into ATP with less variability. This stabilizes the energy environment in which immune and neural processes operate, allowing them to function without compensating for fluctuating supply.

Immune signaling depends on both substrate availability and membrane composition. In a stable system, inflammatory responses are initiated when required and resolved once the objective is achieved. When membrane conditions vary, immune cells interpret signals inconsistently, leading to either exaggerated or insufficient responses. As membrane properties converge, immune recognition, activation, and termination align more closely with input. This allows immune activity to integrate with metabolic state, responding proportionally to actual conditions rather than to distorted signals.

Neural signaling requires precise timing and stable electrical conditions. Membrane integrity determines how well neurons maintain ion gradients and propagate electrical impulses. When permeability is controlled and energy supply is consistent, signal transmission becomes reliable. This allows neural outputs to reflect accurate information about internal and external conditions, coordinating both metabolic and immune responses through central and peripheral pathways.

Cross-system communication becomes more coherent as these conditions stabilize. Hormonal signals that regulate metabolism influence immune activity, and immune mediators affect neural signaling. In a fragmented system, these interactions produce conflicting effects because each system interprets the same signals differently. With restored membrane consistency, these signals produce aligned responses, allowing systems to reinforce rather than disrupt one another.

Feedback loops regain functionality within this integrated environment. Metabolic signals inform immune activity, immune responses influence neural perception, and neural outputs adjust metabolic processes. When outputs are consistent, feedback mechanisms operate with greater accuracy, maintaining balance without excessive oscillation or correction.

Energy allocation becomes coordinated across systems. Rather than competing for limited or inconsistently available resources, metabolic, immune, and neural processes draw from a stable energy supply. This reduces the need for prioritization under stress and allows processes to proceed without disrupting one another.

Temporal alignment improves as activation and termination occur within defined windows. Immune responses begin and resolve in sequence, neural signals propagate with predictable timing, and metabolic transitions occur without overlap or delay. This sequencing depends on consistent membrane conditions that allow each system to operate within shared temporal constraints.

Structural remodeling reinforces integration over time. As membranes across tissues converge toward similar composition, differences in signal interpretation decrease, and system-wide coordination becomes the default state. This does not eliminate specialization but ensures that specialized functions operate within a unified framework.

Reintegration of metabolic, immune, and neural systems therefore emerges from restoring the structural conditions that govern how signals are processed. By aligning membrane properties, stabilizing energy production, and reducing variability in signaling environments, these systems begin to operate as interconnected components of a single network. Their outputs become coordinated because they are derived from the same underlying architecture, allowing the body to respond to inputs as an integrated whole rather than as a set of independent processes.

Stability Across Variable Conditions

A stable system is not defined by constant inputs. It is defined by the ability to maintain consistent output despite changing conditions. Temperature shifts, fluctuations in nutrient availability, variations in activity, and external stressors all alter the environment in which the body operates. Stability emerges when membranes provide a structure that absorbs these changes without allowing them to distort transport, signaling, or energy production. The membrane acts as a buffer, enforcing limits on how much internal conditions can fluctuate in response to external variation.

Mechanical stability is the first requirement. Membranes must maintain their structure under changes in temperature and physical stress. Saturated lipids provide resistance to deformation, while monounsaturated lipids prevent excessive rigidity. Cholesterol adjusts local packing to maintain consistent behavior across a range of conditions. When this balance is present, the membrane does not shift unpredictably in response to environmental changes, and its permeability remains controlled.

Transport processes depend on this consistency. Gradients that drive the movement of ions and substrates must be preserved regardless of external variation. When membrane integrity is stable, passive leakage remains low, and transporters operate under predictable conditions. This allows cells to maintain internal concentrations even when external levels fluctuate, preventing disruption of metabolic processes.

Receptor function must also remain stable across conditions. Changes in temperature, substrate availability, or signaling intensity should not alter the fundamental behavior of receptors. A consistent membrane environment ensures that activation thresholds, clustering behavior, and termination kinetics remain within defined ranges. This allows signals to be interpreted accurately regardless of external variation.

Mitochondrial membranes must preserve gradient integrity under changing demands. Increased activity raises energy requirements, while periods of rest reduce them. A stable inner membrane adjusts output by modulating electron transport without losing containment. Proton leakage remains low, allowing ATP production to scale with demand without introducing variability in efficiency.

Oxidative resistance contributes to stability over time. Exposure to reactive species increases under stress conditions, but membranes that resist oxidation maintain their structure and function. This prevents the accumulation of damage that would otherwise alter permeability and signaling behavior, allowing the system to return to baseline after stress is removed.

Temporal stability depends on the ability to initiate and terminate processes within consistent timeframes. External variation should not extend or shorten these windows unpredictably. When membrane conditions are stable, signaling events begin and end according to internal regulation rather than external disturbance, preserving coordination across systems.

System-wide coordination relies on shared stability across tissues. When membranes in different organs respond similarly to changing conditions, signals produce aligned effects. Hormonal responses remain proportional, neural signaling maintains timing, and immune activity stays within defined limits. This allows the body to adapt without losing coherence.

Energy demand for maintaining stability decreases as structure improves. Fewer resources are required to correct deviations caused by external variation, allowing the system to allocate energy toward adaptation rather than continuous correction.

Stability across variable conditions therefore arises from membranes that maintain consistent physical and electrical properties despite external change. By providing a controlled interface, they ensure that internal processes operate within defined limits, allowing the body to adapt to variation without losing precision, efficiency, or coordination.

Consistent Signaling Across Tissues

System-wide signaling depends on whether different tissues interpret the same input under the same structural conditions. Hormones, neurotransmitters, and immune mediators circulate or propagate with defined concentration and timing, but their effects are determined locally at the membrane. When membrane composition varies, receptors operate under different mechanical and electrical constraints, and identical signals produce divergent outputs. Consistency emerges when membranes across tissues converge toward similar packing, permeability, and domain organization, allowing signals to be translated into aligned responses.

Receptor activation thresholds must match across tissues for signals to produce coordinated effects. Activation depends on controlled receptor mobility and the ability to cluster within organized domains. When membranes differ in fluidity or packing density, some receptors activate at lower concentrations while others require stronger input. This creates uneven responses where certain tissues amplify signals and others dampen them. As membrane properties stabilize, activation thresholds align, and the same signal produces a comparable level of engagement across cell types.

Signal propagation relies on the assembly of downstream components within defined membrane regions. These interactions require consistent spatial organization so that signaling pathways proceed in a predictable sequence. When membrane domains are unstable or vary between tissues, the efficiency of propagation differs, leading to variability in signal strength. Rebuilding domain organization allows signaling complexes to form and function under similar conditions, producing outputs that reflect input rather than local structural differences.

Termination of signaling must occur within similar timeframes to maintain coordination. Prolonged signaling in one tissue and rapid termination in another create temporal mismatch, where processes that should occur in sequence overlap or diverge. Membrane structure influences how quickly receptor complexes disassemble and how effectively baseline conditions are restored. When integrity is consistent, termination kinetics align, allowing signals to begin and end in synchrony across tissues.

Transport of signaling molecules and ions must also operate under uniform conditions. Controlled permeability ensures that gradients are maintained and that movement occurs through regulated pathways. When permeability varies, distribution becomes uneven, altering local concentrations and affecting how signals are perceived. Stabilizing membrane structure reduces this variability, allowing signals to reach tissues with consistent intensity.

Electrical conditions influence signal interpretation, particularly in excitable tissues. Membrane potential depends on maintained ion gradients and selective permeability. When these properties differ, the same signal can produce different electrical responses. Restoring gradient integrity aligns electrical behavior across tissues, supporting consistent signal transmission and response.

Energy availability supports signaling processes at every stage. Activation, propagation, and termination require ATP. When mitochondrial efficiency improves across tissues, energy supply becomes consistent, reducing variability in signaling capacity. This ensures that differences in response are not driven by local energy limitations.

Feedback systems depend on consistent outputs to regulate signaling. When tissues respond differently to the same input, feedback signals become distorted, leading to overcorrection or persistent imbalance. As responses align, feedback loops operate with greater accuracy, maintaining signaling within appropriate ranges.

Remodeling cycles reinforce consistency over time. As stable lipids are incorporated across tissues, membrane properties converge, reducing variability in receptor environments and transport behavior. This gradual alignment produces a system where signals are interpreted under shared conditions.

Consistent signaling across tissues therefore arises from uniform membrane structure that enforces common rules for activation, propagation, and termination. When these conditions are met, signals maintain their meaning as they move through the system, allowing coordinated responses that reflect input rather than local structural variability.

System-Wide Synchronization

Synchronization emerges when multiple systems operate on the same timing, under the same structural constraints, and with access to a consistent energy supply. It is not imposed from a central controller alone. It arises when membranes across tissues enforce similar rules for signal interpretation, transport behavior, and electrical activity. When those rules match, independent processes begin to align in phase, and outputs across the body move together rather than drifting apart.

Temporal alignment begins with signal initiation. Hormonal pulses, neural firing patterns, and immune activation events carry defined timing, but that timing is preserved only if receptor environments respond within the same window. Membrane composition determines how quickly receptors engage and how efficiently signaling complexes assemble. When this varies, identical signals arrive simultaneously but trigger responses at different speeds. As membranes stabilize, initiation kinetics converge, allowing signals to activate tissues in near synchrony.

Propagation timing follows the same constraint. Signals must move through pathways at consistent rates to maintain sequence. This depends on domain organization, ion channel behavior, and maintained gradients. Variability in these properties causes delays or acceleration in specific tissues, disrupting sequence-dependent processes. Uniform membrane structure reduces this variability, allowing signals to propagate through networks with predictable timing.

Termination defines the end of each signaling cycle. If signals persist longer in some tissues than others, processes overlap and interfere. Membrane integrity governs how quickly receptors disengage and how efficiently baseline conditions are restored. When termination kinetics align, signaling events close within the same timeframe, preventing temporal drift between systems.

Energy synchronization supports these processes. ATP production must scale with demand across tissues without introducing delays. When mitochondrial membranes differ in integrity, some cells meet demand quickly while others lag, creating asynchronous behavior. As gradient containment improves and electron leakage decreases, ATP availability becomes more uniform, allowing energy-dependent processes to proceed in parallel.

Electrical synchronization is required for coordinated neural and muscular activity. Membrane potential depends on controlled ion gradients and permeability. When these are stable across tissues, electrical signals maintain consistent amplitude and timing. This allows coordinated firing patterns and reduces noise that would otherwise disrupt signal clarity.

Substrate delivery must also align with timing demands. Transport systems distribute glucose, fatty acids, and other substrates according to gradients and transporter activity. When membrane permeability varies, delivery becomes uneven, causing some tissues to operate ahead of others. Stabilizing transport conditions ensures that substrates arrive in proportion to demand, supporting synchronized activity.

Feedback loops enforce synchronization by adjusting outputs based on system state. These loops depend on accurate, consistent signals from all tissues. When outputs are aligned, feedback maintains timing across systems without excessive correction. When they are not, feedback amplifies variability. Structural consistency allows feedback to stabilize rather than destabilize timing.

Circadian coordination integrates these layers into a repeating temporal framework. Hormonal rhythms, metabolic cycles, and neural activity follow daily patterns that depend on consistent responsiveness across tissues. Membrane stability ensures that these rhythms are expressed uniformly, preventing phase shifts between systems.

Remodeling cycles progressively tighten synchronization. As membranes across tissues converge toward similar composition, variability in timing decreases. Processes that once operated out of phase begin to align, and system-wide behavior becomes predictable.

System-wide synchronization therefore reflects the convergence of timing, structure, and energy across the body. When membranes enforce consistent conditions, signals initiate, propagate, and terminate within shared windows, energy supply matches demand across tissues, and feedback maintains alignment. The result is a system where independent processes operate in coordinated sequence, producing coherent and efficient responses to internal and external inputs.

Chapter 25

Long-Term Structural Maintenance

Long-term stability depends on whether structural conditions are preserved as membranes turn over and environments change. Every cell continuously replaces lipid components through remodeling cycles that respond to substrate availability, oxidative exposure, and metabolic demand. Without control over these inputs, newly built membranes drift away from the properties required for stable signaling and transport. Maintenance is therefore an ongoing process that governs what materials are available for reconstruction, how damage is handled, and whether the system replaces degraded structures with components that restore or further degrade function.

Membrane turnover operates through selective replacement rather than wholesale rebuilding. Individual phospholipids are removed, modified, and reinserted based on the fatty acid pool available at that moment. This means that the composition of circulating and stored lipids directly determines future membrane properties. When stable substrates dominate, replacement cycles gradually reinforce structural integrity. When unstable or oxidized lipids are present, they are incorporated into membranes, introducing variability in packing and increasing susceptibility to further damage. Control of the substrate pool defines the direction of this process.

Oxidative load determines the rate at which structures degrade. Reactive species interact with unsaturated bonds, altering lipid shape and disrupting membrane organization. This increases permeability and destabilizes embedded proteins, forcing higher turnover to maintain function. When oxidative exposure exceeds the system's capacity to repair or replace, damage accumulates faster than it can be resolved. Reducing this load slows degradation, allowing maintenance processes to operate without constant deficit.

Repair systems act on damaged lipids and associated structures to restore function. Enzymatic pathways identify altered components, remove them, and reassemble membranes using available substrates. The effectiveness of these systems depends on both energy availability and the quality of replacement materials. Adequate ATP supports the removal and rebuilding processes, while a stable lipid pool ensures that repaired structures return to a functional state rather than repeating the cycle of instability.

Energy production must remain consistent to sustain maintenance. Remodeling, transport, and repair all require ATP. When mitochondrial efficiency is compromised, energy becomes limited, and maintenance processes are deprioritized. This allows structural degradation to progress, further impairing energy production and creating a reinforcing cycle. Restoring mitochondrial membrane integrity supports the energy supply required to maintain overall structure.

Transport systems influence maintenance by controlling how lipids are distributed and delivered to tissues. Lipoproteins carry triglycerides and phospholipids through circulation, directing them to areas of need. When transport operates efficiently, tissues receive substrates in proportion to demand, supporting uniform maintenance across the system. Disruption in transport leads to uneven distribution, where some tissues rebuild while others degrade.

Hormonal and neural regulation coordinate maintenance activities across tissues. Signals that reflect energy status, nutrient availability, and stress conditions adjust the rate of remodeling and repair. When these signals are interpreted consistently, maintenance processes scale appropriately. Variability in signaling leads to uneven maintenance, reinforcing fragmentation.

Time becomes a defining factor in structural preservation. Membrane replacement occurs over weeks to months depending on tissue type. Short-term changes in input do not immediately translate into structural change, but sustained conditions alter composition progressively. Consistent input of stable substrates allows gradual replacement of unstable components, while continued exposure to damaging conditions prevents convergence toward stability.

Maintenance also requires limiting repeated disruption. Continuous introduction of unstable lipids or persistent oxidative stress forces the system to operate in a reactive state, preventing completion of repair cycles. Removing these inputs allows maintenance to proceed without interruption, enabling the system to reach a steady structural state.

Long-term structural maintenance therefore depends on controlling the inputs that define membrane composition, reducing the forces that drive degradation, and sustaining the energy and signaling conditions required for repair. As these factors align, remodeling cycles reinforce stability rather than erode it, allowing membranes across tissues to maintain consistent properties over time and supporting reliable system-wide function.

Continuous Lipid Turnover and Replacement

Membranes are not static assemblies. Every cell operates a continuous cycle of lipid removal, modification, and reinsertion that reshapes membrane composition over time. This turnover does not occur as a single event but as a distributed process across enzymatic pathways that selectively edit individual phospholipids. Fatty acids are cleaved, exchanged, and re-esterified based on the pool of available substrates, meaning that the circulating and stored lipid environment directly determines what membranes become in the future. Structure is therefore not fixed. It is rewritten continuously through these replacement cycles.

The Lands cycle governs much of this remodeling. Phospholipases remove fatty acids from existing phospholipids, creating lysophospholipids that are then re-acylated with new fatty acids supplied by the cellular pool. This process allows membranes to adapt to changing conditions, but it also makes them vulnerable to the quality of incoming substrates. If stable fatty acids dominate, each cycle reinforces membrane packing and reduces variability. If unstable or oxidized fatty acids are present, they are incorporated into the bilayer, introducing irregular geometry and increasing susceptibility to further damage.

Turnover rates vary across tissues but remain constant enough to ensure that membrane composition reflects long-term inputs rather than short-term fluctuations. Rapidly active tissues such as the liver remodel more quickly, while others change more slowly, but all participate in ongoing replacement. This creates a temporal layer where past inputs persist within structure, gradually displaced as new lipids are incorporated. The system therefore carries a memory of previous conditions until sufficient cycles replace those components.

Oxidative modification accelerates turnover by marking lipids for removal. Reactive species alter double bonds and disrupt membrane organization, triggering enzymatic recognition and extraction. This increases the demand for replacement and shifts the system toward higher throughput. If replacement materials are stable, this process can improve membrane integrity over time. If they are not, turnover becomes a loop where damaged structures are replaced with equally unstable components, preventing convergence toward stability.

Transport systems determine how replacement materials are delivered. Lipoproteins distribute triglycerides, phospholipids, and cholesterol between tissues, directing substrates toward areas of demand. The composition of these carriers reflects dietary input and endogenous synthesis, meaning that systemic lipid distribution shapes local membrane remodeling. Efficient transport allows uniform replacement across tissues, while imbalances create regions where turnover leads to different structural outcomes.

Energy availability constrains the entire process. Lipid remodeling requires ATP for activation, transport, and enzymatic function. When energy supply is consistent, turnover proceeds without interruption, allowing gradual convergence toward stable structure. When energy is limited, incomplete remodeling leads to accumulation of partially processed lipids and inconsistent membrane composition.

Over time, repeated cycles of removal and replacement determine the steady-state composition of membranes. This state is not achieved instantly but emerges from the cumulative effect of thousands of small changes. Each cycle shifts the balance slightly, and sustained conditions drive the system toward a new equilibrium. Stability therefore depends on maintaining inputs that consistently bias these cycles toward structural integrity.

Continuous lipid turnover and replacement define how membranes evolve. By controlling the substrate pool, limiting oxidative disruption, and maintaining energy supply, these cycles can be directed toward building stable, uniform structures. Without that control, the same mechanisms produce variability and instability, embedding those properties into the architecture of the system.

Environmental Pressures and Adaptation

The body does not operate in a fixed environment. Temperature, nutrient availability, light exposure, toxins, and mechanical stress continuously shift the conditions under which cells must maintain structure. Adaptation is the process by which membranes and their associated systems adjust to these pressures without losing functional stability. This adjustment is not abstract. It occurs through changes in lipid composition, protein behavior, and transport dynamics that allow the system to preserve containment, signaling precision, and energy production under altered conditions.

Temperature imposes direct constraints on membrane behavior. Increased temperature accelerates molecular motion, reducing packing density and increasing permeability. Lower temperature produces the opposite effect, tightening packing and restricting movement. Membranes adapt by altering lipid composition to maintain a usable range of fluidity. Saturated lipids resist excessive fluidity under heat, while unsaturated lipids prevent rigidity under cold conditions. Cholesterol acts as a local regulator, inserting between phospholipids to limit extremes in either direction. This balancing process allows membranes to maintain consistent transport and signaling despite external variation.

Nutrient availability shapes the substrate pool used for continuous remodeling. When stable lipid substrates are available, adaptation reinforces structural integrity while adjusting to demand. When unstable or oxidized substrates dominate, adaptation shifts toward maintaining function under compromised conditions, embedding instability into the system. The direction of adaptation therefore depends on the quality of available inputs rather than on the presence of adaptation itself.

Oxidative and chemical exposure introduce structural disruption that must be countered through repair and replacement. Reactive species alter lipid geometry and damage proteins embedded within membranes. In response, cells increase turnover and activate repair pathways to restore function. If the rate of damage exceeds the capacity for repair, membranes accumulate defects that alter permeability and signaling behavior. Adaptation in this context becomes a tradeoff, where the system maintains function at the cost of increased variability and reduced efficiency.

Mechanical stress affects membranes through shear forces, pressure changes, and repeated deformation. Endothelial cells in blood vessels, for example, experience constant fluid shear that influences membrane organization and receptor distribution. Adaptation to these forces involves reinforcing structural elements and adjusting lipid composition to resist deformation while preserving flexibility. This ensures that transport and signaling remain controlled even under continuous physical stress.

Light exposure and circadian input influence membrane-associated processes through timing mechanisms. Hormonal signals that follow daily cycles adjust metabolic activity, repair processes, and energy production. Membranes must respond to these signals within defined temporal windows. Stable membrane conditions allow these rhythms to be expressed consistently, while variability disrupts timing and creates misalignment between systems.

Toxic compounds and xenobiotics introduce additional pressure by interacting with membrane components and altering their behavior. Some compounds insert into lipid bilayers, disrupting packing and increasing permeability. Others generate reactive species that accelerate damage. Adaptation involves both exclusion and repair, limiting the impact of these compounds while restoring structure where disruption occurs. The effectiveness of this response depends on membrane integrity and the availability of resources for repair.

Energy demand fluctuates with activity and stress, requiring membranes to support variable levels of metabolic throughput. Mitochondrial membranes must adjust electron transport rates without losing gradient containment, allowing ATP production to scale with demand. Stable structure enables this flexibility, while compromised membranes leak energy and reduce efficiency under increased load.

Adaptation therefore reflects the ability of membranes to adjust composition and behavior while maintaining core structural properties. These adjustments occur continuously through remodeling cycles that incorporate available substrates and respond to environmental signals. When inputs support stability, adaptation strengthens the system's ability to handle variation. When they do not, adaptation shifts toward maintaining function under degraded conditions, embedding instability into structure.

Environmental pressures do not determine outcomes directly. They define the conditions under which structure must operate. The response of the system depends on whether membranes can adjust while preserving controlled permeability, signaling precision, and energy efficiency. When these properties are maintained, the body adapts without losing coordination. When they are not, adaptation becomes a process of compensation that gradually shifts the system away from stability.

Maintaining Membrane Quality Under Stress

Stress increases the rate at which membranes are challenged and degraded. Elevated temperature, mechanical strain, high metabolic throughput, and reactive species all act on the lipid bilayer, altering packing and increasing permeability. Maintaining membrane quality under these conditions depends on whether the system can limit structural disruption while sustaining the processes that repair and replace damaged components. The outcome is determined by the balance between damage introduction and repair capacity, with membrane composition acting as the primary variable that shifts this balance.

Structural resistance begins with lipid selection. Saturated and monounsaturated fatty acids maintain tighter packing and resist deformation when exposed to thermal or mechanical stress. This reduces the likelihood that membranes will transition into states of excessive fluidity or permeability. Cholesterol reinforces this effect by occupying space between phospholipids, restricting movement under heat while preventing rigid collapse under cooling. When these components dominate, the membrane maintains a consistent barrier even as external conditions fluctuate.

Oxidative stress introduces direct chemical modification of lipids. Reactive species target double bonds, altering molecular geometry and disrupting bilayer organization. This creates defects that increase leakage and interfere with embedded protein function. Membrane quality is preserved when the rate of oxidative damage is limited and when damaged lipids are rapidly identified and removed. Antioxidant systems reduce the frequency of these modifications, while enzymatic repair pathways extract altered lipids and replace them through remodeling cycles. The effectiveness of this process depends on both the availability of stable replacement substrates and the energy required to drive repair.

Turnover rate increases under stress as more lipids require replacement. This raises the demand for transport and remodeling, placing additional load on metabolic systems. If substrate delivery remains consistent and energy supply is sufficient, accelerated turnover can restore membrane integrity without introducing variability. If either is limited, partial repair leads to accumulation of mixed lipid populations, reducing uniformity and increasing susceptibility to further damage.

Protein function within membranes must also be preserved. Receptors, transporters, and channels depend on specific lipid environments to maintain their conformation and activity. Stress-induced changes in membrane composition alter these environments, affecting how proteins behave. Maintaining lipid consistency ensures that these proteins continue to operate within defined parameters, preventing shifts in signaling or transport behavior.

Mitochondrial membranes require particular stability under stress due to increased energy demand. Higher throughput in the electron transport chain elevates the potential for electron leakage and reactive species generation. Cardiolipin composition and membrane packing determine how well the inner membrane contains these processes. When integrity is preserved, ATP production scales without excessive loss. When it is not, energy efficiency declines and oxidative damage increases, reinforcing structural degradation.

Transport systems must continue to regulate substrate and ion movement despite increased stress. Controlled permeability ensures that gradients remain intact, allowing cells to maintain internal conditions even when external pressures fluctuate. Disruption of this control leads to imbalance in ion concentrations and substrate availability, further impairing function.

Temporal control of signaling and repair processes becomes more critical under stress. Activation of protective responses must occur quickly, but termination must also be precise to prevent prolonged disruption. Stable membrane conditions allow these processes to operate within defined timeframes, avoiding overlap or persistence that would increase system strain.

Maintaining membrane quality under stress therefore requires a coordinated response that limits damage, supports rapid and accurate repair, and preserves the structural environment required for protein function and energy production. By controlling lipid composition, sustaining energy supply, and reducing oxidative burden, the system can operate under increased demand without allowing structural degradation to accumulate. This preserves the integrity of membranes across tissues, ensuring that stress does not translate into long-term instability.

Preventing Regression

Structural stability is not permanent once achieved. Membranes remain in a constant state of turnover, and without continued control over inputs and conditions, they drift back toward the same patterns that produced instability. Regression is not a sudden failure. It is a gradual shift in membrane composition, signaling behavior, and transport properties driven by small changes that accumulate over repeated remodeling cycles. Preventing this drift requires maintaining the conditions that originally established stability so that each cycle of replacement reinforces structure instead of eroding it.

The primary control point is the substrate pool. Every remodeling event draws from the available fatty acids and lipid components present in circulation and storage. If this pool shifts toward unstable or oxidized lipids, those materials are incorporated into membranes during normal turnover. The change is incremental but persistent, altering packing density, increasing susceptibility to damage, and disrupting receptor environments. Maintaining a stable substrate pool ensures that replacement cycles continue to produce membranes with consistent mechanical and electrical properties.

Oxidative pressure must remain within the system's capacity to repair. Even with stable substrates, excessive reactive species accelerate damage and increase turnover demands. When the rate of damage rises above repair capacity, incomplete replacement leads to accumulation of defects. Preventing regression therefore involves limiting conditions that elevate oxidative load so that repair systems can operate without deficit.

Energy availability underpins all maintenance processes. Remodeling, transport, and repair require ATP, and any reduction in energy production constrains these functions. When mitochondrial efficiency declines, maintenance becomes inconsistent, allowing degraded structures to persist. Sustaining energy production supports continuous replacement and prevents gaps in maintenance that would otherwise permit regression.

Transport systems must continue to distribute lipids and associated components evenly across tissues. Disruption in transport leads to localized regression, where some areas maintain structure while others degrade. Uniform delivery of substrates allows maintenance processes to proceed consistently, preserving alignment between tissues.

Signaling environments must remain stable to coordinate maintenance across the system. Hormonal and neural inputs regulate the rate of remodeling and repair, adjusting these processes to match conditions. When signals are interpreted consistently, maintenance remains synchronized. Variability in signaling leads to uneven rates of replacement, creating structural divergence that can expand over time.

Exposure patterns determine the long-term direction of remodeling. Short-term deviations have limited impact, but repeated or sustained exposure to destabilizing inputs shifts the equilibrium of membrane composition. Preventing regression requires maintaining conditions that favor stability over extended periods so that cumulative effects continue to move the system toward consistent structure.

Feedback mechanisms help maintain stability when outputs accurately reflect internal state. As membranes remain consistent, feedback loops regulate processes without overcorrection, preserving balance. If regression begins, distorted outputs disrupt feedback, allowing further drift. Maintaining accurate signaling supports these regulatory systems in preventing deviation.

Time remains the governing factor. Structural stability is preserved through repeated cycles that replace any emerging inconsistencies with stable components. When conditions remain controlled, each cycle reinforces the desired state, reducing the likelihood of drift. If conditions change, the same cycles begin to move the system in the opposite direction.

Preventing regression therefore depends on sustaining the inputs and conditions that maintain membrane integrity. By controlling substrate quality, limiting oxidative disruption, ensuring energy availability, and preserving coordinated signaling, the system continues to rebuild itself in a stable configuration. Without these controls, continuous turnover becomes the mechanism through which instability re-emerges, gradually shifting the architecture away from the state required for consistent function.

CONCLUSION

THE RETURN TO STRUCTURE

Biological function does not originate from isolated pathways or individual molecules acting in abstraction. It emerges from the physical organization of the system, where membranes define boundaries, control exchange, and establish the conditions under which all processes operate. When this structure is stable, signaling is precise, transport is controlled, and energy production proceeds without loss. When it degrades, the same processes persist but produce inconsistent and often conflicting outputs. The difference is not in the presence of activity but in the conditions that shape how that activity unfolds.

The collapse into calorie-based thinking removed structure from the model and replaced it with accounting. Energy intake and expenditure became the focus, while the architecture that determines how energy is used was ignored. This shift explains why interventions built on energy balance alone fail to produce consistent outcomes. Without stable membranes, inputs are processed under variable conditions, leading to unpredictable behavior. Restoring structure returns the model to the level where outcomes are determined, allowing the system to operate under defined constraints.

Membranes function as the governing layer that integrates all systems. They regulate permeability, maintain gradients, and provide the environment in which receptors, transporters, and enzymes operate. Lipid composition determines how these functions behave, influencing mechanical stability, electrical properties, and signaling dynamics. This places lipids at the center of biological organization, not as passive energy sources but as structural components that define system behavior over time.

The body maintains itself through continuous turnover, replacing lipid components based on available substrates and environmental conditions. This process allows adaptation but also introduces vulnerability. Without control over inputs, remodeling cycles incorporate instability into the structure, gradually altering function. With consistent input of stable substrates and reduced disruption, the same cycles reinforce integrity, aligning membranes across tissues and restoring coordinated behavior.

System-wide coordination depends on shared structural conditions. Metabolic, immune, and neural systems communicate through signals that require consistent interpretation. When membranes differ, these systems operate under conflicting rules, producing fragmented outputs. As membrane properties converge, signaling aligns, energy production stabilizes, and feedback mechanisms regain accuracy. The body shifts from a state of compensation to one of coordination, where processes reinforce rather than interfere with one another.

Long-term maintenance ensures that this state persists. Continuous control of substrate quality, oxidative load, and energy availability allows remodeling cycles to preserve structure rather than erode it. Environmental pressures remain, but the system adapts to them without losing stability because the underlying architecture is maintained. This prevents regression and supports consistent function across varying conditions.

The return to structure reframes biology at its foundation. It moves the focus from inputs measured in isolation to the physical system that determines how those inputs are processed. By maintaining membrane integrity and controlling the conditions that shape remodeling, the body operates with predictable, efficient, and coordinated behavior. Outcomes follow from structure, and when structure is restored, the system returns to a state where its functions align with the demands placed upon it.

Biology as a Material System

Biology operates through physical materials organized into functional structures, not through abstract pathways detached from their environment. Cells are constructed from lipids, proteins, and aqueous compartments arranged in a way that constrains how molecules move, interact, and transform. Every outcome in the body reflects how these materials are assembled and how they behave under given conditions. Signals, reactions, and energy flow all depend on this arrangement. Without the correct material properties, the same inputs produce different outputs because the system itself has changed.

Membranes define the primary material boundary of the system. They separate internal conditions from the external environment and regulate what crosses that boundary. The lipid composition of these membranes determines permeability, mechanical strength, and electrical behavior. A tightly packed membrane limits uncontrolled movement, preserving gradients that drive transport and energy production. A disordered membrane allows leakage, dissipating gradients and altering how signals are interpreted. This boundary is not passive. It is the interface that shapes all internal activity.

Proteins operate within this material framework and depend on it for proper function. Receptors require specific lipid environments to maintain their conformation and to cluster with associated signaling components. Transporters depend on membrane thickness and fluidity to cycle between states that move substrates across the bilayer. Enzymes embedded in membranes interact with lipids that influence their activity and stability. When the surrounding material changes, protein behavior changes with it, even if the protein itself remains structurally intact.

Energy production is constrained by material properties. Mitochondrial membranes must contain proton gradients to drive ATP synthesis. This containment depends on lipid composition, particularly the presence of cardiolipin and tightly packed phospholipids that reduce leakage. When the material fails to maintain this barrier, energy dissipates as heat rather than being captured as ATP. The efficiency of energy conversion therefore reflects the integrity of the membrane rather than the availability of substrates alone.

Signaling systems rely on spatial organization within membranes. Lipid microdomains create regions where specific proteins concentrate, allowing signals to be initiated and propagated efficiently. These domains depend on lipid interactions that define their size, stability, and composition. When the material is consistent, signaling pathways operate with defined timing and strength. When it is not, signals become diffuse or exaggerated, leading to variability in response.

Transport processes are governed by gradients that exist because of material boundaries. Ion concentrations, substrate levels, and electrical potential differences are maintained by limiting uncontrolled exchange. Membrane composition determines how well these gradients are preserved. Stable materials support controlled transport through channels and carriers, while unstable materials allow passive leakage that disrupts distribution and forces compensatory activity.

Adaptation occurs through changes in material composition. Cells adjust lipid content, protein expression, and structural organization in response to environmental conditions. These changes are incorporated through continuous turnover, meaning that the material state of the system reflects cumulative inputs over time. Adaptation therefore modifies structure first, and function follows as a consequence of that structural shift.

Damage is also material in nature. Oxidation, mechanical stress, and chemical interactions alter the physical properties of lipids and proteins, disrupting their organization. Repair involves removing damaged components and replacing them with new materials that restore the original structure. The success of this process depends on both the availability of appropriate substrates and the energy required to perform the replacement.

Viewing biology as a material system places emphasis on what the body is made of and how those materials are arranged. It explains why identical biochemical pathways can produce different outcomes under different structural conditions and why long-term inputs shape function by altering composition. When the material properties of the system are stable, processes operate within defined limits and produce consistent results. When they are not, variability emerges from the structure itself, influencing every level of function.

Structure as the Driver of All Outcomes

Outcomes in biology follow from structure because every process is constrained by the physical conditions in which it occurs. Membranes define those conditions by setting permeability, organizing proteins, and maintaining gradients that enable transport and energy production. When this structure is consistent, inputs are processed within defined limits and produce predictable results. When it varies, the same inputs lead to different outputs because the underlying environment has changed. Function does not drift on its own. It follows the state of the material that supports it.

Signaling behavior reflects membrane organization. Receptors activate, cluster, and terminate based on the local lipid environment that controls their mobility and interaction with downstream components. When membranes maintain stable packing and domain structure, signals are interpreted with consistent thresholds and timing. Variability in composition alters these parameters, shifting activation sensitivity and prolonging or shortening responses. The signal itself remains unchanged, but its effect diverges because the structure that receives it has shifted.

Transport depends on structural containment. Gradients of ions and substrates exist only when membranes restrict uncontrolled movement. These gradients drive the entry and exit of materials through regulated pathways, allowing cells to maintain internal conditions distinct from their surroundings. When membrane integrity declines, leakage increases and gradients weaken, forcing compensatory mechanisms to restore balance. This alters distribution and increases energy demand, changing how substrates are delivered and used across the system.

Energy production is determined by the ability of mitochondrial membranes to contain and utilize proton gradients. The electron transport chain generates a difference in charge and concentration that must be preserved to produce ATP. Structural defects in the membrane allow protons to return without driving ATP synthesis, reducing efficiency and increasing heat loss. Energy availability therefore depends on the physical integrity of the membrane rather than on substrate supply alone.

Immune activity is shaped by structural recognition and signaling. Membranes present molecular patterns that determine how immune cells identify targets and initiate responses. Lipid mediators derived from membrane components control the intensity and duration of these responses. When structure is stable, recognition and resolution proceed in sequence. When it is not, signaling becomes prolonged or misdirected, leading to incomplete resolution or inappropriate activation.

Hormonal responses depend on receptor environments and transport conditions. Hormones circulate with defined concentration and timing, but their effects are determined by how receptors respond within each tissue. Membrane composition sets the conditions for this response, influencing sensitivity and signal propagation. Structural consistency allows hormonal signals to produce coordinated effects across tissues, while variability creates divergence in response.

Neural function relies on controlled electrical properties of membranes. Ion gradients and channel behavior determine how signals are generated and transmitted. Stable membrane structure preserves these gradients and supports consistent conduction. Structural disruption alters electrical behavior, introducing variability in signal transmission and timing.

All systems converge on the same dependency. The body operates as a network of processes that require stable boundaries, controlled exchange, and consistent signaling environments. These requirements are met through membrane structure, which integrates lipid composition, protein organization, and energy dynamics into a single framework. Changes in this framework propagate through every level of function, altering outcomes without changing the inputs themselves.

Structure therefore acts as the governing layer of biology. It determines how signals are interpreted, how substrates are distributed, and how energy is produced and used. By maintaining membrane integrity and controlling the conditions that shape it, the system operates within predictable limits. When structure degrades, variability emerges, and outcomes become inconsistent. The direction of change is set not by the processes themselves but by the material state in which those processes occur.

Lipids as the Foundation of Control

Control in biological systems does not originate from signaling molecules alone. It emerges from the material that defines how those signals are received, transmitted, and terminated. Lipids form that material. They construct the membranes that determine permeability, organize proteins into functional arrangements, and establish the electrical and mechanical conditions required for coordinated activity. Without stable lipid structure, control is lost even when signaling inputs remain unchanged, because the system no longer interprets those inputs in a consistent way.

Membrane permeability is the first layer of control. Lipid packing determines how easily ions and molecules cross the bilayer outside of regulated pathways. Tightly packed membranes restrict passive movement, preserving gradients that drive transport and electrical activity. When packing loosens, leakage increases, gradients weaken, and control shifts from regulated transporters to uncontrolled diffusion. This changes how substrates are distributed and how signals propagate, introducing variability that the system must compensate for through increased energy expenditure.

Spatial organization of proteins depends on lipid composition. Receptors, channels, and enzymes are not randomly distributed. They localize within specific lipid environments that support their function. Cholesterol and sphingolipids create ordered regions where signaling complexes assemble, allowing rapid and coordinated activation. The surrounding lipid matrix determines how these domains form, how stable they remain, and how quickly they disperse after signaling is complete. Changes in lipid composition alter this organization, affecting both the strength and timing of signal transmission.

Electrical control is also lipid-dependent. Membrane potential arises from the separation of charge across the bilayer, maintained by ion gradients and selective permeability. Lipids influence both the ability to sustain these gradients and the behavior of embedded ion channels. Stable membranes support consistent electrical properties, allowing predictable signal generation and conduction. Structural disruption alters ion leakage and channel function, changing how electrical signals are initiated and propagated.

Energy production is governed by lipid structure within mitochondria. The inner mitochondrial membrane must contain proton gradients to convert electron flow into ATP. Cardiolipin and tightly packed phospholipids create the conditions required for this containment. When lipid composition shifts, proton leakage increases, reducing the efficiency of energy conversion. This affects every process that depends on ATP, linking energy availability directly to membrane integrity.

Lipid-derived molecules extend control into signaling pathways. Fatty acids released from membranes serve as precursors for mediators that regulate inflammation, vascular tone, and immune activity. The types of lipids present determine which mediators are produced and how long they persist. This ties signaling outcomes to the structural composition of membranes, making lipid balance a determinant of system behavior rather than a passive background factor.

Adaptation and regulation occur through continuous lipid turnover. Remodeling cycles replace existing fatty acids with those available in the cellular pool, gradually altering membrane composition. This process allows the system to adjust to environmental conditions, but it also means that long-term inputs shape control mechanisms over time. Stable inputs reinforce consistent control, while unstable inputs introduce variability that propagates through signaling, transport, and energy systems.

Feedback mechanisms depend on lipid-defined conditions to operate correctly. Signals generated in response to changes in system state must be interpreted consistently across tissues to maintain balance. When lipid composition diverges, feedback becomes inaccurate, leading to overcorrection or persistent imbalance. Maintaining lipid integrity ensures that these regulatory loops function within expected parameters.

Lipids therefore provide the foundation of control by defining the environment in which all biological processes occur. They regulate what enters and leaves cells, organize the components that transmit signals, and maintain the conditions required for energy production. By shaping these core functions, lipids determine how the system behaves as a whole. Control is not imposed on the system from above. It is built into the structure of the membranes that govern every interaction within it.

Stability as the Basis of Health

Health reflects the ability of the system to produce consistent outputs under changing conditions. This consistency depends on structural stability, where membranes maintain controlled permeability, organized signaling environments, and contained energy gradients despite fluctuations in temperature, nutrient availability, and external stress. When structure is stable, processes operate within defined limits and return to baseline after perturbation. When it is not, variability accumulates, and the system shifts into continuous correction rather than controlled function.

Membrane stability preserves gradients that define internal conditions. Ion concentrations, electrical potential, and substrate distribution all depend on the ability to restrict uncontrolled exchange. Stable lipid packing maintains these gradients, allowing transport systems to operate predictably. When membranes lose integrity, leakage increases, gradients weaken, and cells must expend additional energy to restore balance. This alters distribution patterns and reduces efficiency, affecting every downstream process that depends on controlled internal conditions.

Signaling stability emerges from consistent receptor environments. Activation thresholds, clustering behavior, and termination kinetics depend on membrane composition. When these properties remain within a defined range, signals are interpreted with precision, producing proportional responses. Structural variability shifts these parameters, leading to exaggerated or diminished signaling that disrupts coordination between tissues. Stability ensures that signals maintain their meaning as they move through the system.

Energy stability is determined by mitochondrial membrane integrity. ATP production requires containment of proton gradients and efficient electron transport. Stable membranes support this process, allowing energy output to match demand without excessive loss. Structural disruption increases proton leakage and reactive species generation, reducing efficiency and creating variability in energy availability. Consistent energy supply supports all maintenance, repair, and functional processes.

Temporal stability allows processes to occur within defined windows. Activation and termination of signaling, repair cycles, and metabolic transitions depend on predictable timing. Stable membranes enable these processes to begin and end without distortion, preserving sequence and coordination. When timing varies between tissues, processes overlap or diverge, leading to interference and inefficiency.

Resistance to stress is a consequence of structural stability. Mechanical forces, oxidative exposure, and metabolic demand all challenge membrane integrity. When membranes resist deformation and damage, the system can absorb these stresses without altering core function. This reduces the need for compensatory responses and allows rapid return to baseline conditions once stress is removed.

System-wide coordination depends on shared stability across tissues. When membranes in different organs maintain similar properties, signals produce aligned effects, and feedback mechanisms operate accurately. This allows metabolic, immune, and neural systems to function as an integrated network. Variability in structure disrupts this alignment, creating fragmentation where systems operate under different constraints.

Long-term stability is maintained through continuous turnover that replaces degraded components with stable ones. Each remodeling cycle either reinforces or erodes structural integrity depending on substrate availability and environmental conditions. Sustained input of stable lipids and controlled oxidative load allow these cycles to converge toward consistent membrane composition, preserving function over time.

Health therefore arises from the maintenance of stable structural conditions that govern all biological processes. By preserving membrane integrity, supporting energy production, and ensuring consistent signaling environments, the system operates with predictable and coordinated behavior. Stability allows the body to adapt to variation without losing control, making it the underlying basis from which reliable function emerges.

Made in the USA
Monee, IL
05 November 2026

67914370R00164